Introduction to Epidemiology

Second edition

Ilona Carneiro and
Natasha Howard

Lucianne Bailey, Katerina Vardulaki,
Julia Langham and Daniel Chandramohan

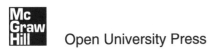
McGraw Hill

Open University Press

Open University Press
McGraw-Hill Education
McGraw-Hill House
Shoppenhangers Road
Maidenhead
Berkshire
England
SL6 2QL

email: enquiries@openup.co.uk
world wide web: www.openup.co.uk

and Two Penn Plaza, New York, NY 10121-2289, USA

First published 2005
Reprinted 2010
First published in this second edition 2011

A catalogue record of this book is available from the British Library

ISBN-13: 978-0-33-524461-4
ISBN-10: 0-33-524461-0
eISBN: 978-0-33-524462-1

Library of Congress Cataloging-in-Publication Data
CIP data applied for

Typeset by RefineCatch Limited, Bungay, Suffolk
Printed in the UK by Bell & Bain Ltd, Glasgow.

Fictitious names of companies, products, people, characters and/or data that may be used
herein (in case studies or in examples) are not intended to represent any real individual,
company, product or event.

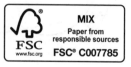

To Ariana and Alesia Marin Carneiro

and

Alya Howard

Contents

List of figures

List of tables

Preface

This book represents a thorough revision of the first edition. The structure of the book has been changed to help the flow of learning. Key concepts of chance, bias, confounding and causality are now introduced earlier to help student understanding. The concept of standardization is introduced later to improve the pace at which new material is covered. The chapters on risk assessment and screening methods have been combined as both relate to preventive strategies. A new chapter on study design has been written to bring together issues common to all epidemiological studies, and may be used as a quick reference when developing a study protocol. Finally, the chapter on surveillance includes a new section on the application of epidemiology for monitoring and evaluation of health programmes.

We have aimed to clarify the terminology and concepts covered in the original version, and have revised the examples and activities to cover a wider range of more contemporary health issues, with additional focus on developing countries. The number of activities has been increased and we have moved the feedback to the end of the chapters for this new edition to help readers test their understanding of the material more effectively. New material includes: measuring the secondary attack rate for outbreak investigation, the use of case-control studies for genetic epidemiology and plausibility designs for intervention studies.

Acknowledgements

The authors wish to thank colleagues who have developed the original lectures and teaching materials at the London School of Hygiene & Tropical Medicine: Lucianne Bailey, Katerina Vardulaki, Julia Langham and Daniel Chandramahon who wrote the first edition; Ros Plowman, and Nicki Thorogood (Series Editors) and Julia Langham, Daniel Chandramohan and John Carneiro for reviewing chapters in the 2nd edition. We are grateful to the students of the Public Health Distance Learning course for their challenging questions that have helped to improve the material, especially Peter Simpson, Dina Khan, Aaron Hawkins, Anita Dubey and Julie Nabweteme who piloted various chapters.

Overview of the book

Introduction

This book is intended for self-directed learning. It provides a summary of the main concepts and methods of epidemiology as a foundation for further study. It will also introduce more advanced epidemiological and statistical concepts to broaden understanding. After completing the book, you should be able to apply basic epidemiological methods and critically interpret the epidemiological findings of others.

Why study epidemiology?

Epidemiology is integral to public health. Whether your interest is in clinical or public health medicine, the study of epidemiology is key to improving health. Neither clinical nor public health practice can be based on experience alone; they must be based on scientific evidence. Understanding the appropriateness of different research methods is essential to critical appraisal of the evidence presented in scientific literature. The ability to distinguish between strong and poor evidence is fundamental to promoting evidence-based healthcare. This ability is important for all those who work in health-related areas, including health economists, health policy analysts, and health services managers. Epidemiology is central to clinical research, disease prevention, health promotion, health protection and health services research.

Epidemiology offers rigorous methods to study the distribution, causation and prevention of poor health in populations. It enables a better understanding of health and the factors that influence it at individual and population-levels. Epidemiological methods are also used to investigate the usefulness of preventive and therapeutic interventions, and the coverage of healthcare services. The purpose of epidemiology is to use these methods and the resulting data to improve health and survival.

Structure of the book

This book is structured around the basic concepts, practices and applications of epidemiology and uses the conceptual framework of the basic epidemiology module taught face-to-face at the London School of Hygiene & Tropical Medicine. It is based on materials presented in lectures and seminars, which have been adapted for distance learning.

Chapters 1–4 discuss the principles of epidemiology and introduce strategies for measuring the frequency of health outcomes, associations and impact of exposures, and evaluating whether an association is causal. Chapters 5–10 focus on practical aspects of epidemiological research, including issues of study design and data collection and the strengths and weaknesses of each of the principal epidemiological study designs. Chapters 11–12 consider the application of epidemiology for prevention strategies, and surveillance, monitoring and evaluation.

Each chapter includes:

- an overview
- a list of learning objectives
- a range of activities
- a concluding summary
- feedback on the activities

In each chapter, some words are presented in italics to add *emphasis*. Words presented in **bold** are described in the Glossary on p.171. You may find the index at the end of the book useful for finding terms that you are unsure of or wish to review.

Guidance notes for activities

We recommend that you attempt the activities as they appear in the text, and refer back to the preceding explanatory text if you find a question unclear or difficult. You should complete the whole of each activity before reading the relevant feedback at the end of each chapter, as this will help you assess your understanding of the material presented. As is usual in epidemiology, most activities will include numerical calculations and require interpretation of results.

The required mathematical skills will be fairly basic, but may require the use of a calculator. Proportions (e.g. 0.20) can be presented as percentages by multiplying by 100 (i.e. $0.20 \times 100 = 20\%$). Except for percentages, answers should generally be rounded to two decimal places (e.g. 0.148 reported as 0.15), and statistical probability values are usually rounded to three decimal places (e.g. 0.0025 reported as $p = 0.003$). It is important not to round numbers until the very end of a mathematical operation, to avoid the accumulation of error due to rounding and remain as precise as possible.

SECTION I

Key principles of epidemiology

Principles of epidemiology

1

Overview

Epidemiology is the cornerstone of public health. It employs rigorous methods and a quantitative approach to study the health of *populations* rather than individuals. Epidemiological methods are used to identify the causes of poor health, measure the strength of association between causes and outcomes, evaluate interventions and monitor changes in population health over time. The study of epidemiology provides the evidence-base for appropriate public health policy, planning and practice. This chapter provides an introduction to the key approaches of epidemiological research.

Learning objectives

When you have completed this chapter you should be able to:

- describe the key aspects of epidemiology
- discuss the complex factors involved in the study of causality
- identify the basic study designs used in epidemiology
- recognize the role of epidemiology in society.

What is epidemiology?

Epidemiology is *the study* of the distribution and determinants of health states or events in specified populations, and *the application* of this study to control health problems (adapted from Porta and International Epidemiological Association, 2008). Health states or events usually refer to infection, illness, disability, or death but may equally be used to refer to a positive outcome (e.g. survival). Epidemiological studies describe the distribution of these health **outcomes** in terms of frequency and pattern. The *frequency* is the number of occurrences of an outcome within a given time period, and the *pattern* refers to the occurrence of the outcome by time, place and personal or population characteristics. Determinants influence the frequency and pattern of health outcomes and are known as **risk factors** or **protective factors**, depending on whether they result in a negative or positive health outcome respectively.

Epidemiological research also involves the testing of preventive interventions (e.g. vaccines, improved hygiene) and therapeutic interventions (e.g. medicines, surgery) to improve health and survival. An intervention may be evaluated either under ideal (research-controlled) conditions to assess its **efficacy** or through a routine delivery system to assess its **effectiveness**.

After collecting epidemiological evidence, its application to improve health is a natural progression. Identification of risk factors and protective interventions, and quantification of their effects are key to informing action. Knowledge of the distribution and time-trends of outcomes, risk factors, and intervention coverage may be used for advocacy, for health promotion, and to inform public health policy and practice.

The study of epidemiology

The two main approaches to epidemiological study are **descriptive** and **analytical** (Figure 1.1). Descriptive epidemiology may provide information on the distribution of health outcomes by age, population type, geography or over time. Sources of descriptive data include routine monitoring such as registers of births and deaths, notification systems of specific diseases or adverse treatment reactions, and hospital or clinic records. Population censuses may also provide data on births, deaths, and a variety of risk factors (e.g. age, gender), and there is an overlap with demography (i.e. research on changes in the size, structure and distribution of human populations). Population health surveys evolved from censuses and provide information on the use of health services, coverage of interventions and the frequency of specific outcomes.

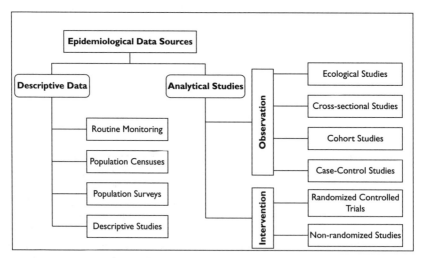

Figure 1.1 Main sources of epidemiological data

Source: Ilona Carneiro.

Activity 1.1

Figure 1.2 shows a declining trend in the incidence of rheumatic fever in Denmark since 1900. Briefly describe what this might suggest.

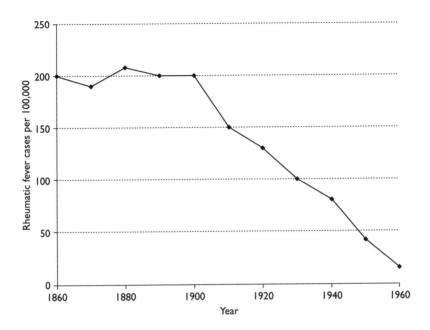

Figure 1.2 Incidence of rheumatic fever in Denmark, 1862–1962

Source: Taranta and Markowitz (1989) – graph re-drawn by Ilona Carneiro from Beaglehole et al. (1993).

Cause and effect

Analytical epidemiology aims to investigate which factors may be responsible for increasing or decreasing the probability ('risk') of an outcome. Identifying the cause of an outcome is not always simple, and can be described in terms of **sufficient cause** and **component causes**. Sufficient cause refers to a factor or set of factors that inevitably produces the outcome. The factors that form a sufficient cause are called component causes. Some component causes are essential for the outcome to occur: tuberculosis cannot occur without *Mycobacterium tuberculosis*, and this is known as a **necessary cause**. However, some people may be infected with *M. tuberculosis* without developing tuberculosis, because other components such as immune status and concurrent infections (e.g. HIV) will determine their susceptibility to the disease.

A single necessary cause is rarely sufficient to cause the outcome. While this may make epidemiological investigation of causality more difficult to untangle, it works to our advantage in public health, as it means that there are often several points at which we can intervene to reduce the likelihood of an outcome. Necessary causes may be:

1 infectious agents such as viruses, bacteria or parasites;
2 environmental agents such as sun-rays or allergens (e.g. pollen, dust-mites);
3 industrial agents such as chemicals (e.g. nicotine) or radiation (e.g. mobile phones);
4 genetic factors such as chromosomal abnormalities;
5 physical factors such as violence or car accidents;
6 psychological factors such as stress or abuse.

Component causes may influence an individual's contact or response to a necessary cause. Environmental factors tend to affect contact and may be physical (e.g. climate, altitude), biological (e.g. vectors that transmit an agent) or structural (e.g. crowding, sanitation). Human factors affect both contact and response, and include age, sex, ethnicity, behaviour, genetics, and nutritional and immunological status. These environmental and human factors also interact, making the whole process even more complex. For example, people living in conditions of poor sanitation will have greater contact with the polio virus because transmission is mainly via faecal contamination. Children will be at greater risk of infection than adults because of their poorer sanitary practices and also because of their lack of natural immunity or incomplete immunization.

As you may have realized, depending on the perspective we take, a cause can also be considered as an outcome for the purpose of epidemiological investigation. For example, human immunodeficiency virus (HIV) is a necessary cause of acquired immunodeficiency syndrome (AIDS). However, we might then want to consider HIV infection as an outcome, and identify the necessary cause as unprotected sex with an infected individual, or contact with contaminated needles. This leads us to consider other risk factors that might increase the likelihood of HIV infection: multiple sexual partners, sharing of intravenous drug needles or poor safety practices in health facilities. However, while these risk factors can be component causes, they are not necessarily causal. A person may become infected through only one sexual contact, while another person with multiple sexual partners may not become infected at all.

Relating a causative agent or risk factor – from here on termed **exposure** – to an outcome of interest is known as inferring **causality**. For an association to be causal, the exposure must occur before the outcome. Other factors that support a causal relationship include a dose–response relationship, the strength of the association seen, a plausible biological mechanism of action, and reproducibility of the result. These and other factors that support causality will be discussed in more detail in Chapter 4.

Alternative explanations

Analytical methods may confirm an association between an exposure and outcome, but causality can only be inferred if alternative explanations, namely chance, bias and confounding, have been accounted for. **Chance** is the possibility that there is **random error** and is usually reduced by increasing **sample size**, using **random selection** (observational studies) or **randomization** (intervention studies). **Bias** refers to systematic differences between comparison groups, which may misrepresent the association being investigated. **Confounding** is caused when another factor, independently associated with both the outcome and exposure of interest, influences the association being investigated. These alternative explanations for an apparent association between an outcome and exposure, and the challenges of inferring causality, will be discussed in Chapter 4.

Analytical study designs

The main approach to investigating causal relationships is through analytical studies. An epidemiological investigation starts with the development of a **hypothesis**, which takes the form of a proposed association that can be tested. For example, 'smokers are at a higher risk of lung cancer'. An analytical study will then aim to find out whether there is sufficient or insufficient evidence to support this hypothesis.

Analytical epidemiology takes two forms: observation or intervention (Figure 1.1). An **observational study** aims to compare the frequency of the outcome in groups or individuals with and without the exposure of interest. An intervention study is effectively an experiment, and therefore restricted to evaluating the effect of reducing a risk factor or increasing a protective factor on the frequency of an outcome. Five study designs form the core of epidemiological research and these will be considered in more detail in Chapters 6–10:

1 **Ecological studies** consider populations of individuals and aim to relate the total frequency of an outcome to an average level of exposure by population group. For example, differences in alcohol consumption and incidence of breast cancer by country.
2 **Cross-sectional studies** collect data on outcome and exposure at one point in time from a random sample of study **subjects**. For example, prevalence of HIV in relation to male circumcision.
3 **Cohort studies** compare individuals with recorded differences in exposure to measure the occurrence over time of the outcome in relation to exposure. For example, incidence of cervical cancer in women with and without human papillomavirus infection.
4 **Case-control studies** identify individuals with and without the outcome, and examine whether they differ in relation to previous exposure. For example, mobile telephone use among people with brain tumours compared to those without brain tumours.
5 **Intervention studies** allocate a protective factor to individuals or groups, and compare the frequency of the outcome in those exposed with those unexposed. For example, the incidence of malaria among children given an insecticide-treated mosquito net, compared with those given an untreated mosquito net. Intervention studies may be randomized or non-randomized.

The application of epidemiology

The data and relationships identified through epidemiological study may be used in various ways. Descriptive epidemiological methods enable health professionals to identify the actual and potential health problems in a population. The burden of health outcomes or associated risk factors can be quantified, related to existing health services, and tracked to predict changes over time. An overview of the health issues affecting a population, and more importantly the relative distribution of these outcomes, enables priorities to be set and programmes to be planned. For example, Figure 1.3 shows that the incidence of road traffic deaths among children was estimated to be greater in Africa than in Europe for 2004, highlighting the need for relevant interventions in Africa.

Once a risk factor has been identified through analytical studies, health promotion activities may be developed to reduce exposure to the outcome at the individual level (e.g. encouraging smokers to stop smoking through education and support programmes) or population level (e.g. banning smoking in public places). Screening programmes may be implemented to increase early diagnosis and appropriate treatment (e.g. recommended mammograms for all women over 50 years old, who are at greater risk of breast cancer than younger women).

Monitoring and evaluation of health programmes are necessary to assess whether an implemented intervention is safe and effective under routine conditions, and whether

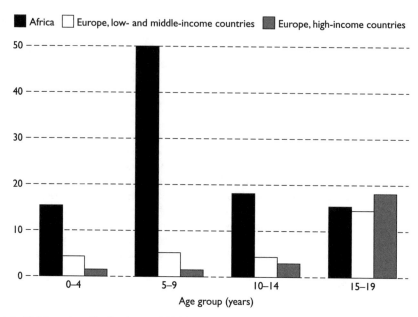

Figure 1.3 Child road-traffic deaths per 100,000 population
Source: WHO (2008).

this can be maintained over time. This may take the form of routine surveillance for the outcome (e.g. number of measles cases), or monitoring of specific programmatic indicators (e.g. number of children receiving three doses of measles vaccine).

Activities 1.2–1.5

To help you put some of these epidemiological ideas into context, you will now look at a famous example from the nineteenth century.

John Snow (1813–58), a distinguished physician and considered one of the fathers of epidemiology, is best known for his studies of cholera outbreaks in London between 1848–49 and in 1854 (Snow 1936). These are the first documented epidemiological investigations. Activities 1.2–1.5 use John Snow's cholera studies to illustrate the epidemiological approach, from descriptive epidemiology and hypothesis generation (1.2), to hypothesis testing and refinement (1.3–1.4), and application of epidemiological data (1.5). After attempting each activity you should refer to the feedback at the end of the chapter to prepare you for the next activity. Feedback does not provide the only true answers, as there are many accurate ways to answer these questions.

Cholera periodically swept across Europe during the nineteenth century. Cholera was characterized by profuse painless diarrhoea and clear fluid vomit that caused rapid dehydration, but the cause was unknown. After a severe epidemic in London in 1832, cholera reappeared in 1848. The first definite case was a seaman, newly arrived from Hamburg where cholera was prevalent. He died a few hours after the onset of symptoms on 22 September 1848 in a hotel near the River Thames. The next case was a lodger in the same room, who developed cholera symptoms on 30 September 1848. During the epidemic, approximately 15,000 deaths were recorded. Cholera mortality in this epidemic was particularly high in residential areas downstream from the hotel, and decreased progressively upstream.

Microorganisms had not yet been discovered and one of the popular beliefs about disease causation was the 'miasma' theory – that breathing bad air caused disease. John Snow had previously documented several instances in which people had come into contact with cases of cholera and developed the disease within a few days. While investigating several case series of cholera, he made the following observations:

- Cholera was more readily transmitted within poor households and to those who had handled a case of cholera.
- Miners had suffered more than any other occupation.
- Almost no doctor who attended to cholera cases or conducted post-mortems had developed cholera.
- Most cases of cholera developed within 24–48 hours after contact with a case of cholera.
- Cholera was characterized by profuse painless diarrhoea and often proceeded with so little feeling of general illness that patients did not consider themselves in danger, or seek advice, until the illness was far advanced.

Activity 1.2

1 If you were a doctor in Snow's time, list what hypotheses you might generate about cholera transmission from these observations.
2 Describe how Snow might have interpreted his observations to oppose the 'miasma theory' and support alternative hypotheses such as those in question 1.
3 Identify what the most plausible explanations are for the observed association between elevation of residential area and level of mortality from cholera.

Activity 1.3

During the nineteenth century, private companies that obtained water directly from the river Thames supplied the drinking water in London. Each company had its own network of pipes. In some areas these networks overlapped and different companies could supply houses along a single street. The Southwark and Vauxhall (S&V) Company and the Lambeth Company were the two major water suppliers to the cholera-affected areas during the epidemics that John Snow investigated.

Between 1849 and 1853, when London was free of cholera, the Lambeth Company moved its water source upstream to an area outside London, while the S&V Company continued to draw water from a downstream source in London. Snow collected data on the number of houses supplied by the S&V Company and the Lambeth Company. When the cholera epidemic recurred in London in 1854, he collected data on sources of water for households of those who died of cholera. Table 1.1 shows the number of cholera deaths per 10,000 households, stratified by water source, during the first seven weeks of the epidemic.

1 Do the data presented in Table 1.1 support Snow's hypothesis that cholera is transmitted through water? Give reasons for your answer.

Table 1.1 Water sources and cholera mortality in London, 9 July to 26 August 1854

Source of water	Total number of households	Number of cholera deaths	Deaths per 10,000 houses
S&V Company	40,046	1,263	315
Lambeth Company	26,107	98	37
Rest of London	256,423	1,422	59

Source: Adapted from John Snow (1936).

2 Are these data adequate to conclude that cholera mortality is higher in houses supplied by the S&V Company than in houses supplied by the Lambeth Company? Give reasons for your answer.

3 What further questions might you ask before reaching any conclusions based on these data?

Activity 1.4

Snow investigated a severe outbreak of cholera in the Soho area of London. He collected house addresses of all 616 recorded cholera deaths between 19 August and 30 September 1854. From these data he produced a map showing the distribution of cholera deaths (bars) and positions of the water pumps (filled-circles) used by Soho households (Figure 1.4). This is known as a 'spot map'.

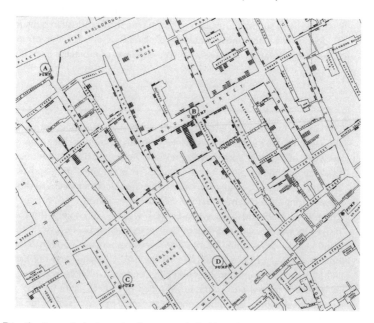

Figure 1.4 Distribution of cholera deaths around Golden Square, London, August–September 1854 presented in a 'spot map'

Source: John Snow (1936).

1 Describe the distribution of cholera deaths in relation to the position of water pumps in Figure 1.4.
2 What might explain the differences in the distribution of deaths around water pumps A, B, C and D?
3 Can you conclude that water from a particular pump was the source of the cholera epidemic? Give reasons for your answer.
4 What further information do you need?

Activity 1.5

Snow discovered that a brewery was located in the two blocks with no cholera deaths with a deep well on the premises. The brewery workers and people living nearby collected water from the brewery well. Additionally, brewery workers had a daily quota of malt liquor. This information convinced Snow that pump B was the source of the cholera. He persuaded the local authorities to remove the pump-handle, preventing further use of the pump after the 8th September.

The dates of onset of symptoms of the 616 fatal cases of cholera recorded between 19 August and 30 September are shown in Figure 1.5.

1 Describe what the graph in Figure 1.5 shows.
2 Did removal of pump B end the cholera epidemic? Explain your answer.
3 What other factors might explain why the epidemic stopped?

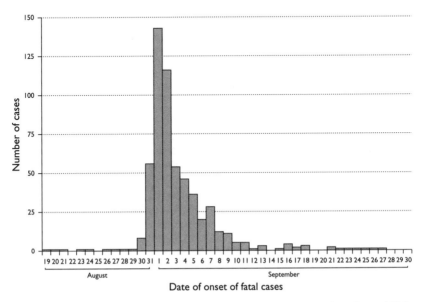

Figure 1.5 Distribution of cases of cholera by date of onset (based on data from Snow, 1936)

Source: Drawn by Ilona Carneiro using data from John Snow (1936).

Conclusion

Epidemiology includes both a scientific approach (evidenced-based medicine) and a societal perspective (population-based studies and solutions) to health. You have been introduced to several new concepts and terms that are key to the understanding of epidemiology: descriptive epidemiology, inferring causality, analytical study designs, interpretation of results and the applications of epidemiology. These issues are fundamental for those involved in clinical and public health, and will be discussed further in subsequent chapters.

References

Beaglehole R, Bonita R and Kjellstrom T (1993) *Basic Epidemiology*, Geneva: World Health Organization.
Porta MS and International Epidemiological Association (eds) (2008) *A Dictionary of Epidemiology*, Oxford: Oxford University Press.
Snow J (1936) *Snow on Cholera (being a reprint of two papers)*, London: Oxford University Press.
Taranta A and Markowitz M (1989) *Rheumatic fever: a guide to its recognition, prevention and cure*. 2nd edn. Lancaster: Kluwer Academic Publishers.
World Health Organization (2008) *The World Health Report 2008: Primary Health Care – Now More Than Ever*, Geneva: World Health Organization.

Feedback for activities

Activity 1.1

The graph in Figure 1.2 shows that the incidence of rheumatic fever drops particularly sharply after 1900, having been relatively steady for the previous 40 years. This suggests that some event might have triggered the decline in the incidence of rheumatic fever around 1900.

Rheumatic fever is caused by haemolytic streptococcal upper respiratory tract infection, which is associated with poverty and overcrowding. Therefore, it is reasonable to suggest that the decline in rheumatic fever was the result of improvements in socioeconomic conditions in Denmark that occurred at the beginning of the twentieth century.

Activity 1.2

1 You might have listed some or all of the hypotheses that Snow developed. Based on his observations, Snow generated the following hypotheses on the mode of transmission of cholera:
   • Cholera can be transmitted from the sick to the healthy.
   • Cholera is caused by some material (Snow called it 'morbid matter') that can increase and multiply in the body of the person it attacks.
   • The causative agent must be introduced into the alimentary canal by swallowing.
   • The causative agent may be transmitted through water from the sick to the healthy.
2 To dispute the miasma theory, Snow argued that:
   • The risk of transmission of cholera was high in miners and people of low socioeconomic status because these groups had poor hygiene practices and were, therefore, more likely to have contact with faecal matter from cholera patients than those of higher socioeconomic status.

- Few doctors developed cholera because they washed their hands after seeing each cholera patient.
- If transmission were through the air or via a vector, the disease would have been transmitted from cholera patients to more doctors.
- Thus, the disease was most likely caused by some causative agent transmitted by direct contact.

3 The observed association between higher elevation of residential area and lower mortality from cholera could support the theory of bad air causing cholera. However, as Snow argued, the water downstream of the initial cases was more likely to be polluted with sewage than the water upstream. Thus, the increased risk of cholera transmission in the areas downstream also supported his theory that the causative agent was most probably transmitted through water.

Activity 1.3

1 Yes, these data support Snow's hypothesis that cholera is transmitted through water, but they do not prove it. For example, no information on other possible modes of transmission is included.

2 The risk of cholera death was 315/10,000 in houses supplied by the S&V Company, 38/10,000 in households supplied by Lambeth Company, and 55/10,000 in houses supplied by other sources. These data suggest that the risk of cholera death was 8–9 times higher (315/38) in households supplied by the S&V Company than in households supplied by the Lambeth Company. However, they do not prove causality and are not adequate to make firm conclusions that cholera mortality is higher in households supplied by the S&V Company.

3 Before reaching any conclusions, you would want to consider whether the number of people per household, their socioeconomic status, and other potential factors associated with the risk of transmission of cholera are comparable between these two populations. For example, the S&V Company might have supplied water to multiple-occupancy buildings while Lambeth supplied individual family houses. If this were the case, then the risk of cholera death per house between the two populations would not be comparable since the average number of people per house would differ between them. Since the S&V Company was drawing water from downstream, it is possible that households supplied by the company would have been in downstream areas and might be poorer than households upstream. Thus, although these data appear to support Snow's hypothesis, more information is needed to be convincing.

Activity 1.4

1 Figure 1.4 shows that there was a cluster (collection) of many deaths around pump B (the Broad Street pump), very few deaths near pumps A and D, and almost no deaths around pump C.

2 If water from all the pumps was the source of cholera, there would probably have been similar numbers of deaths around each pump rather than more around pump B. However, it is possible that people did not drink the water from pumps A, C and D due to bad taste, smell, or inconvenience, or that the water from these pumps might not have carried the cholera causative agent.

3 While pump B has the greatest spatial clustering of cholera deaths and might have been the source, this is not sufficient to conclude that pump B was the source of

cholera. Two blocks of buildings very close to pump B did not have a single death from cholera.

4 More information is needed to explain the absence of deaths in the two blocks nearby before implicating the water from pump B as the source of the epidemic. For example, if it could be shown that there was no death in these blocks for reasons such as:

- No one lived there.
- Inhabitants had alternative sources of water.
- Inhabitants had some kind of protection against cholera.

Activity 1.5

1 There appears to have been a low background number of cases (zero or one case per day) before 30th August. There was an explosive rise in the number of cases over three days, which decreased to previous levels after 12 days. The most likely explanation for the sudden rise in the number of cholera deaths would be exposure of the population to a causal agent from a common source.

2 It is unlikely that removal of the pump-handle from pump B stopped the epidemic, because the number of cholera deaths had already dropped to almost the background level by the time the pump-handle was removed. However, removing the pump-handle B may have prevented another outbreak of cholera if pump B still contained the causal agent and was available for use.

3 There are several possible explanations for the end of the epidemic:

- People who lived in the epidemic area might have moved elsewhere due to fear of contracting cholera.
- All **susceptible** people (those who had no form of immunity to cholera and were therefore at-risk of infection) might have been exposed within a short time, leaving very few susceptible individuals.
- The amount of causal agent in the water could have reduced.

Vibrio cholera, the bacterium that causes cholera, was identified by Robert Koch in 1883, several decades after Snow identified appropriate preventive measures from his epidemiological investigations:

I feel confident, however, that by attending the above mentioned precautions (personal hygiene, boiling soiled bedclothes of patients, isolation and quarantine, improved waste disposal, drainage, provision of clear water), which I consider to be based on correct knowledge of the cause of cholera, this disease may be rendered extremely rare, if indeed it may not be altogether banished from civilized countries.

(Snow 1936)

Measuring the frequency of outcomes $\boxed{2}$

Overview

The occurrence of health outcomes (i.e. infection, illness, disability and death) will vary between populations, geographical areas and over time. Epidemiological studies quantify the **frequency** of health outcomes, which is the number of occurrences in a defined population over a defined time-period. In this chapter you are introduced to the epidemiological measures used to determine the frequency of outcomes: prevalence, risk (including attack rates), odds and incidence rates.

Learning objectives

When you have completed this chapter you should be able to:

- identify and define the four common frequency measures: prevalence, risk, odds and incidence rate
- calculate each of these frequency measures
- recognise the use of attack rates in the investigation of outbreaks
- estimate person-time at risk.

Defining a case

To measure the frequency of an outcome in a population, it is first necessary to have a clear definition or description to identify the outcome of interest. In some situations the outcome is obvious (e.g. all cause death), but often, standardized criteria are needed (e.g. severe anaemia may be defined as haemoglobin less than 5 grams per decilitre). Individuals with the outcome of interest are often referred to as 'cases'. The criteria used to define them form the **case definition**, which may not be clinically defined. The outcome may refer to an event such as a car accident rather than an illness. A 'case' may occur only once per individual (e.g. death), more than once (e.g. pregnancy), or frequently (e.g. diarrhoeal disease). Epidemiologists count cases using clinical assessments, diagnostic tests, registry or clinic record entries, observation, or even self-reporting in population surveys.

Knowing the number of cases is not enough to allow any comparison or association to be made. If you were told that there were 75 cases of tuberculosis in village A and only 25 cases in village B, you might be tempted to conclude that tuberculosis was more common in village A than in village B. However, without knowing how many people live in each village, this comparison is impossible to make. Once cases have been defined and counted, it is necessary to count the number of individuals in the population from which cases were identified and the time-period in which the cases occurred, to calculate frequency.

Measuring disease frequency

The most common measures of disease frequency (i.e. prevalence, risk, odds, incidence rate) vary according to how cases and time-period are considered. We will use the analogy of a children's game of musical chairs, where everybody dances while the music is played, and chairs are removed at regular intervals when the music stops. Those left without a chair on which to sit have to stand to one side until the game finishes. We can explain the measures of frequency as follows, where the outcome is 'sitting on a chair':

1 *Prevalence* counts the number of children sitting at a specific time point (e.g. at 11:30a.m.), compared with the total participants in the game (standing and sitting) at that same time point.
2 *Risk* counts those sitting after a specified time-period (e.g. after 10 minutes), compared with the total participants at the start of the game.
3 *Odds* counts those sitting after a specified time-period (e.g. after 10 minutes), compared with those standing after the same time-period.
4 *Incidence rate* counts those sitting at any point during the game and the total time that each individual participates, allowing for children who join the game late or leave early.

Prevalence

Prevalence is the number of *existing* cases in a defined population at a defined point in time divided by the total number of people in that population at the same point in time:

$$\text{Prevalence} = \frac{\textbf{Number of cases at one time point}}{\substack{\textbf{Total number of individuals in the defined population} \\ \textbf{at same time point}}}$$

Prevalence is a proportion and can never be greater than one. It is dimensionless, meaning that it has no units, so the term 'prevalence rate' is incorrect. Prevalence is usually presented as a percentage by multiplying the proportion by 100. Prevalence is sometimes referred to as **point prevalence** to distinguish it from **period prevalence**. Period prevalence refers to the number of existing cases identified during a specified, usually short, period divided by the total number of people in that population during the same period.

The prevalence of an outcome may be measured during population surveys or cross-sectional studies. Prevalence is useful to rapidly assess the frequency of an outcome in a community. For example, in a cross-sectional survey of 200 boys aged 5–10 years old in a low-income setting, 60 were found to be stunted, i.e. had a height-for-age lower than the average. The prevalence of stunting in this group would be calculated as 60 ÷ 200 = 0.30, which would be presented as 0.3 × 100 = 30% of young boys in this population being stunted (an indicator of chronic malnutrition) at the time of the survey.

Incidence

Incidence is the frequency of *new* ('incident') cases in a defined population during a specified time-period. Incidence may be measured in ecological or cohort studies. There are three different ways of considering incidence: risk, odds and incidence rate.

Risk

Risk is also known as **cumulative incidence** because it refers to the total number of new cases in a defined 'population at risk' over a specified period of time:

$$\text{Risk} = \frac{\textbf{Number of new cases in a specified time-period}}{\textbf{Total number of individuals at risk in the population at the start of that time-period}}$$

This measure can be interpreted as the likelihood ('risk') that an individual will develop an outcome during the specified time-period, and the 'population at risk' excludes existing ('prevalent') cases. Risk is also a dimensionless proportion, so can never be greater than one and has no units. However, its value can increase with the duration of the time-period under consideration, making it essential to specify the period at risk. For example, if a group of 100 people were studied for a year, and 75 had caught at least one cold during that year, we could say that the risk of catching a cold was 75 ÷ 100 = 0.75 or 75% in that year in that group. However, the result would be interpreted differently if 100 people had been studied for six months and 75 had caught at least one cold during this six-month period; it would have to be specified as a 75% risk over 6 months.

A specific form of risk used in disease outbreak settings is called the **secondary attack rate**. This is a misnomer, as it is a proportion and not a rate (see below), but the term is commonly accepted. The secondary attack rate is calculated as the number of new cases among contacts of a primary case in a specified period of time:

$$\text{Secondary attack rate} = \frac{\textbf{Number of new cases among contacts in a specified time-period}}{\textbf{Total number of contacts of a primary case in that time-period}}$$

This can be interpreted as the 'risk' that a contact of a case will develop the outcome during the specified time-period. The total number of contacts is often estimated from the household members of primary cases, but may also include school or workplace contacts. For example, if eight children developed varicella (chicken pox) in an outbreak at a school, and five out of a total of 15 siblings developed varicella in the subsequent two weeks, we could estimate the secondary attack rate, or risk of developing varicella among household contacts, as 5 ÷ 15 = 0.33 or 33% in this two-week time-period.

Odds

Odds is a different way of representing risk, and is calculated as the number of *new* cases divided by the number of individuals still at risk after a specified time- period:

$$\text{Odds} = \frac{\textbf{Number of new cases in a specified time-period}}{\textbf{Number who did not become a case during that time-period}}$$

The odds is actually a ratio of two proportions and can be greater than one. It is the ratio of the 'risk' that an individual develops the outcome during a specified time-period, to the 'risk' that the individual does not develop the outcome during that same time-period. Below you can see how this simplifies mathematically to the equation given above, as the denominator (total number at risk) is the same for both outcomes, and cancels-out:

$$\text{Odds} = \frac{\text{Cases}}{\text{Total}} \div \frac{\text{Non-cases}}{\text{Total}} = \frac{\text{Cases}}{\text{Total}} \times \frac{\text{Total}}{\text{Non-cases}} = \frac{\text{Cases}}{\text{Non-cases}}$$

In the example, in which 75 people in a group of 100 caught a cold during a particular year, the odds of catching a cold would be calculated as $75 \div 25 = 3$. The odds of catching a cold would be 3 to 1, sometimes reported as 3:1, so that a person in that group would be three times more likely to catch a cold as not to catch a cold during that year.

Incidence rate and person-time at risk

Both risk and odds assume that the population at risk is followed over a specified time-period, and that all those who are included at the beginning of the time-period are counted at the end of the time-period. This is called a *closed* population. However, you might want to look at incidence in a *dynamic* or *open* population, in which people enter and exit the population at risk at different points and are therefore at risk for different lengths of time. Once the outcome has occurred, the individual will either no longer be at risk or, if the outcome can recur, there will be some interval of time before the individual is once more considered at risk. Therefore, instead of counting the total number of people at the start of the study, the time that each individual is at risk is calculated. This is known as the **person-time at risk** and is illustrated in Figure 2.1. People may start and stop being at risk at different times, due to births and deaths, immigration, acquiring the outcome, leaving the study population before the end (known as 'lost to follow-up'), or reaching the end of the observation period.

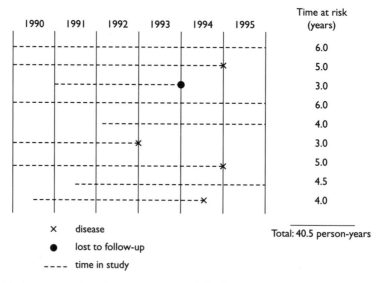

Figure 2.1 Graphical representation of person-time at risk for 9 study participants during a 6-year study period

Source: Bailey et al. (2005).

The **incidence rate** allows us to account for variation in time at risk, and is calculated as the number of new cases divided by the total person-time at risk:

$$\text{Incidence rate} = \frac{\textbf{Number of new cases in a specified time-period}}{\textbf{Total person} - \textbf{time at risk during that time-period}}$$

This measure is a rate and is reported as the number of new cases per person-time at risk. It is essential to specify the time units, for example person-days, person-months, person-years, or more frequently 1,000 person-years at risk.

In Figure 2.1, the incidence rate is obtained by dividing the total number of cases by the total number of person-years at risk. Four people became cases during the study, so the incidence rate is $4 \div 40.5 = 0.099$ cases per person-year at risk, or 99 cases per 1,000 person-years at risk (to avoid the use of too many decimal places).

In registry data or very large studies it might be difficult to know the exact person-time at risk for each individual in the population. In this situation, the population at the mid-point of the time-period of interest is multiplied by the period of time under consideration to give an estimate of the person-time at risk, so long as the population size does not change substantially over the study period. For example, data from a cancer registry (a record of all cancer cases notified by doctors) found 750 cases of breast cancer in a region of a politically-stable country between 2005 and 2010. The population of that region was recorded from a census to be 10,130 in 2007–2008. The person-time at risk is estimated as the mid-period population multiplied by the five-year period at risk. The incidence is calculated as $750 \div (10,130 \times 5) = 750 \div 50,650 = 0.015$ per person-year at risk, or to reduce loss of precision due to rounding, $0.0148 \times 1,000 = 14.8$ cases of breast cancer per 1,000 person-years at risk between 2005–2010.

Activity 2.1

Investigators were asked to determine the prevalence of malaria cases in two villages in rural Southeast Asia. There were 500 people (210 men and 290 women) in the two villages. Investigators spent a couple of days in November testing everyone in the villages for malaria, using rapid diagnostic tests (which detect malaria parasite-specific proteins in blood). Investigators found that 62 men and 22 women tested positive for malaria.

1 Write a simple case definition investigators could have used in this study.
2 Define the study population.
3 Based on your case definition and study population, what is the malaria prevalence among men and among women in the villages?

Activity 2.2

An outbreak of human monkeypox, a relatively rare orthopox viral disease similar to but milder than smallpox, was detected in a forested province of the Democratic Republic of Congo (DRC). Investigators found 5 secondary cases of monkeypox among 37 house-hold contacts of a 9-year-old boy who was the first reported to have become infected.

1 Assuming all household contacts are equally at risk, what is the secondary attack rate among household contacts?
2 Data from previous outbreaks suggests that prior smallpox vaccination confers 85% protection from monkeypox. If all household contacts had been vaccinated against smallpox, how would this change your secondary attack rate calculation?

Activity 2.3

Investigation of an outbreak of measles, in remote District X, found 12 cases of measles had occurred among 350 children attending a local school over a one-month period. Each infected child came from a different household. The total number of additional children (i.e. household child contacts) in the 12 affected households was 67. Ten children in the affected households had previously had measles, while 20 children were reported to have received at least one dose of measles vaccine. However, immunization records were poor and many children had not been fully immunized. One month (i.e. approximately two incubation periods) later, four more children in the 12 affected households also developed measles.

1 What was the risk of measles in the school during the initial one-month period?
2 What is the secondary attack rate among household child contacts of the 12 children?
3 What does this tell us?

Activity 2.4

Investigators conducted a survey of intestinal worm infestation among 1,000 adoles-cent agricultural workers in Country Y. They found 620 adolescents were infested with one or more type of worm. After treating all adolescents found positive, investigators returned six months later and tested all 1,000 adolescents again. This time they found 390 adolescents infested.

1 Calculate the prevalence of worm infestation among adolescents in the first survey.
2 Calculate the risk and the odds of worm infestation among adolescents during the six-month study period.
3 What is the incidence rate of worm infestation among adolescents during the six-month study period?

Activity 2.5

One thousand men working in factory A were screened for HIV on 1 January 2010 and 50 of them were found to be HIV-positive. When the screening was repeated on the same 1,000 men on 1 January 2011, 62 men were positive, including the 50 men who were positive on the first screening. Nobody had died or been lost to follow-up.

1 What is the prevalence of HIV in men working in factory A on 1 January 2010, and on 1 January 2011?
2 What is the annual risk of developing HIV infection in men working in factory A during 2010?
3 What are the odds of developing HIV infection in men working in factory A during 2010?

Activity 2.6

One thousand men in factory B were screened for HIV on 1 January 2010 and 50 men were found to be HIV-positive. All of these men were tested for HIV at the end of each month until 31 December 2010. Twelve men became HIV-positive during this period, while the remaining 938 men were still HIV-negative by 31 December 2010. Figure 2.2 shows when these 12 men became HIV-positive. Nobody died or was lost to follow-up during this period.

1 What is the total number of person-months at risk of HIV infection observed in this study?
2 What is the incidence rate of HIV infection among men working in factory B?
3 What are the odds of becoming infected with HIV in the first six months of 2010 compared with becoming infected in the last six months of 2010?

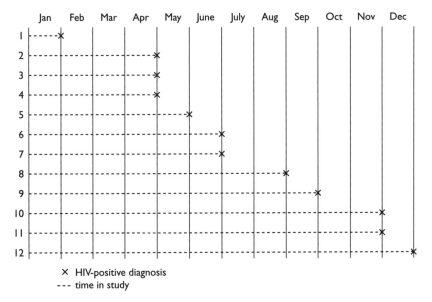

Figure 2.2 Person-months at risk of HIV in factory B in 2010

Source: Bailey et al. (2005).

Conclusion

You have been introduced to the measures of prevalence and incidence (risk, odds and incidence rate) that are used to quantify the occurrence of an outcome in a defined population. These epidemiological measures of frequency help in assessing the public health importance of an outcome and planning appropriate health services. These measures also form the basis of analytical studies to investigate the association between exposures and outcomes.

Reference

Bailey L, Vardulaki K, Langham J and Chandramohan D (2005) *Introduction to Epidemiology* 1st edn. Maidenhead: Open University Press.

Feedback for activities

Activity 2.1

1 You may have said that cases could have been defined as those individuals resident in one of the two villages who tested positive for malaria by rapid diagnostic test during the two days in November.

2 The study population includes all 500 individuals in the two study villages. There were 210 men and 290 women.

3 The number of prevalent cases among men is 62. There were 210 men tested. Therefore, the prevalence of malaria in men is $62/210 \times 100 = 0.295 \times 100 = 30\%$. The number of prevalent cases among women is 22. There were 290 women tested. Therefore, the prevalence of malaria in women is $22/290 \times 100 = 0.076 \times 100 = 7.6\%$.

Activity 2.2

1 The number of cases of monkeypox among secondary contacts = 5. The total number of secondary household contacts = 37. Therefore, the secondary attack rate = $5 \div 37 \times 100 = 0.135 \times 100 = 13.5\%$.

2 The total number of secondary household contacts estimated to be unprotected by vaccination = $37 - (37 \times 0.85) = 37 - 31.45 = 5.55$ (i.e. 6) unprotected household contacts. The number of cases of monkeypox among secondary contacts = 5

To calculate the secondary attack rate in this scenario we divide the number of cases among secondary contacts by the number of unprotected household contacts = $5 \div 5.55 \times 100 = 0.90 \times 100 = 90\%$. This would indicate a dramatically more virulent monkeypox strain than did the first scenario.

Activity 2.3

1 The number of cases of measles among children at the school = 12. The total number of children at the school = 350. Therefore, the incidence risk = $12 \div 350 \times 100 = 0.34 \times 100 = 3\%$.

2 The number of secondary cases of measles among household child contacts of the 12 children is 4. The total number of children at risk in the affected households = (total number of contacts – previous measles cases) = $67 - 10 = 57$. Therefore, the secondary attack rate among unvaccinated child contacts is the number of cases among household child contacts out of those child contacts who are actually known to be at risk (i.e. not already a case) = $4 \div 57 \times 100 = 0.0702 \times 100 = 7\%$.

   In reality, there may be a higher number of contacts immune to measles through vaccination or prior disease.

3 An initial risk of (3%) and a secondary attack rate of (7%) indicate that the outbreak is increasing or that transmission is more efficient within households than within the school. As measles can be prevented by vaccination, the increase in cases suggests that vaccination coverage is insufficient and a mass measles vaccination campaign should be organized.

Activity 2.4

1 The number of prevalent cases in the first survey = 620. The total number of adolescents tested is 1,000. Therefore, the prevalence of infestation among adolescents in the first survey is $(620 \div 1,000) \times 100 = 0.62 \times 100 = 62\%$.

2 The number of incident cases in the second survey = 390. The total number of adolescents tested is 1,000. Therefore, the risk of infestation among adolescents during the six-month period is (390 ÷ 1,000) × 100 = 0.39 × 100 = 39%. The number of cases in the second survey = 390. The number of adolescents who are not cases = 1,000 – 390 = 610. Therefore, the odds of infestation among adolescents during the six-month period are (390 ÷ 610) × 100 = 0.64 × 100 = 64%.

3 The number of incident cases in the second survey = 390. As we do not know how many months each adolescent contributed to person-time at risk, we need to use the mid-period population, calculated as the average of the population at start and end of the study (i.e. (1,000 + 1,000)/2 = 1,000, thus 1,000 × 6 = 6,000 person-months), and assume that the adolescents did not leave the study area for significant periods during the six-month period. Therefore, the incidence rate of infestation among adolescents is estimated as (390 ÷ 6,000) × 1000 = 0.065 × 1000 = 65 per 1,000 person-months.

Activity 2.5

1 The number of prevalent cases at 1 January 2010 = 50. The total number of individuals tested in this population on 1 January 2010 = 1,000. Therefore, the prevalence at 1 January 2010 = (50 ÷ 1,000) × 100 = 5%.

  The number of prevalent cases at 1 January 2011 is 62. The total number of individuals tested in this population at 1 January 2011 is 1000. Therefore, prevalence at 1 January 2011 = (62 ÷ 1000) × 100 = 6.2%.

2 The number of incident (new) cases in 2010 is 62 – 50 = 12. The number of individuals at risk of HIV infection on 1 January 2010 = 1000 – 50 = 950. Therefore, the annual risk of developing HIV infection in 2010 = (12 ÷ 950) × 100 = 1.26%.

  The 50 men who were HIV-positive on 1 January 2010 are not included in the denominator because HIV-positive individuals do not become HIV-negative. Therefore those who were HIV-positive on 1 January 2010 were not at risk of developing HIV infection during 2010.

3 The number of incident cases during 2010 is 62 – 50 = 12. The number of individuals at risk of HIV infection in 2010 who did not become infected is 950 – 12 = 938. Therefore, the odds of developing HIV infection in 2010 = 12 ÷ 938 × 100 = 1.28%.

Activity 2.6

1 To calculate total person-months at risk, add total person-months contributed by men who remained HIV-negative and total person-months contributed while they were HIV-negative by men who subsequently became infected (as men who were already infected at the beginning of study do not contribute any person-months at risk).

  Person-months at risk for men who remained HIV-negative throughout the study period = 938 × 12 = 11,256. Person-months at risk for the 12 men infected during the study period = 1 + (3 × 4) + 5 + (2 × 6) + 8 + 9 + (2 × 11) + 12 = 81. Therefore, total person-months at risk during the study period = 11,256 + 81 = 11,337.

  Another way to look at this is that, as we do not know when exactly these men became infected, it would be more accurate to assume that 'on average' they contributed only 0.5 months at risk for the month prior to testing HIV-positive. Using this approach, total person-months at risk for the 12 men infected during the study period = 0.5 + (3 × 3.5) + 4.5 + (2 × 5.5) + 7.5 + 8.5 + (2 × 10.5) + 11.5 = 75.

Using this approach, total person-months at risk during the study period would be 11,256 + 75 = 11,331. In this particular example, as the overall person-time at risk is large, this will not make a difference to our estimate of incidence rate below.

2 To calculate an incidence rate, select an appropriate unit of person-time at risk for the denominator. In this example, person-months is an appropriate unit, as time at risk is already segmented into months and person-months contributed can be calculated easily from Figure 2.2.

Total number of incident cases = 12. Total person-months = 11,337. Therefore, incidence rate = (12 ÷ 11,337) × 1,000 = 1.06 per 1,000 person-months.

3 To calculate odds, divide the number of men who became HIV-positive in the first half of 2010 by the number who did not (i.e. who became positive in the second half of 2010).

Number of men who became HIV-positive in the first six months of 2010 = 7. Number of men who did not become HIV-positive during first six months = 5. Therefore, *of those who became HIV-positive in 2010*, the odds of becoming HIV-positive in the first 6 months = 7/5 = 1.4. In other words, among those who became HIV-positive in 2010, the odds of becoming infected in the first half of the year were 40% higher (difference from an odds of 1, i.e. 1.4 − 1.0 = 0.4 or 40%) than the odds of becoming infected in the second half of the year.

Measures of association and impact 3

Overview

Analytical epidemiology is concerned with quantifying the association between an exposure and an outcome, to establish causal relationships and identify effective interventions. This chapter presents different ways to measure the association between an exposure and an outcome, and you will be introduced to several new terms and formulae.

First, *relative* measures of association use the frequency measures you learned about in the previous chapter to compare the frequency of outcomes in different exposure groups. These take the form of ratios: *prevalence* ratio, *risk* ratio, *odds* ratio and *incidence rate* ratio.

Second, you will be introduced to measures of impact: attributable risk, attributable fraction, population attributable risk and population attributable fraction. Evidence of an association between a modifiable exposure and an outcome can be used to assess potential impact, i.e. the additional burden of outcome due to the exposure that may be prevented if that exposure is removed.

Learning objectives

When you have completed this chapter you should be able to:

- recognize different measures of association: prevalence ratio, risk ratio, odds ratio and incidence rate ratio
- recognize different measures of impact: attributable risk, attributable fraction, population attributable risk, population attributable fraction
- define, calculate and interpret each of these measures of association and impact
- identify the appropriate measure of association for a given epidemiological objective.

Relative measures of association

Relative measures estimate the extent (*strength*) of an association between an exposure and an outcome. The relative measures that use ratios to compare the frequency of an outcome are prevalence ratio, risk ratio, odds ratio and incidence rate ratio. These are collectively referred to as measures of **relative risk**. However, it is good practice to refer to specific relative risk measures by name, to avoid confusing the term 'relative risk' with the specific 'risk ratio' measure.

Relative risk measures indicate how much more likely it is that an exposed individual will develop the outcome compared with an unexposed individual. If the relative risk is greater than one, then exposed individuals are at greater risk. If the relative risk equals one, there is no difference in risk between the exposed and unexposed. If the relative risk is less than one, exposed individuals are at a lower risk, and the exposure can be called a protective factor. Table 3.1 illustrates the standard format for presenting comparative data in an epidemiological study and will be used to clarify the differences between the different measures of relative risk.

Table 3.1 Standard cross-tabulation (2 × 2 table) of outcome by exposure

		Outcome		
		Yes	No	Total
Exposure	Exposed	a	b	a + b
	Unexposed	c	d	c + d
	Total	a + c	b + d	a + b + c + d

Source: Ilona Carneiro.

Prevalence ratio

The **prevalence ratio** can be calculated from cross-sectional studies or population surveys. In practice, this is the least useful of the measures described in this chapter as the exposure and the prevalence of the outcome are measured at the same time point, making it difficult to infer causality. We cannot distinguish whether an associated factor has caused the outcome to occur or has simply caused it to persist as a prevalent case. It is calculated as the prevalence in exposed individuals divided by the prevalence in unexposed individuals:

$$\text{Prevalence ratio} = \frac{\text{Prevalence of outcome in the exposed group}}{\text{Prevalence of outcome in the unexposed group}}$$

If Table 3.1 is taken to represent the number of existing cases by exposure group detected at one time point, the overall prevalence of the outcome in the sample population is calculated as $(a+c)/(a+b+c+d)$. The prevalence in the exposed group is given by $a/(a + b)$ and the prevalence in the unexposed group is given by $c/(c + d)$, so the prevalence ratio is calculated as:

$$\text{Prevalence ratio} = \frac{a/(a + b)}{c/(c + d)}$$

It is not necessary to know the actual number of cases or the total number of individuals, as long as the prevalence in each exposure group is known. For example, you are told that the prevalence of obesity, defined as body mass index greater than 30 kg/m^2, is 20% in people reporting that they do less than 2 hours of exercise per week, and 10% in those reporting that they do at least 2 hours of exercise per week. The prevalence ratio for obesity can be calculated as $0.10 \div 0.20 = 0.50$ in those 'exposed' to at least 2 hours of exercise per week. This can be interpreted as exposed individuals being 0.50 times or half as likely to be obese as those unexposed. The ratio can also be inverted as $0.20 \div 0.10 = 2.0$, such that those 'exposed' to less than 2 hours of exercise are twice as likely to be obese as those unexposed.

Risk ratio

The **risk ratio** can be calculated from ecological, cohort or intervention studies. The risk ratio is calculated as the risk (cumulative incidence) of the outcome in the exposed group divided by the risk (cumulative incidence) of the outcome in the unexposed group:

$$\textbf{Risk ratio} = \frac{\textbf{Risk of outcome in the exposed group}}{\textbf{Risk of outcome in the unexposed group}}$$

If Table 3.1 is taken to represent the number of new (incident) cases by exposure group detected during a defined time-period, the overall risk of the outcome in the sample population can be calculated as $(a+c)/(a+b+c+d)$. You will see that these equations are identical to those for prevalence, because risk is also a proportion as discussed in the previous chapter, but are applied to incident cases. The risk in the exposed group is given by $a/(a + b)$ and the risk in the unexposed group is given by $c/(c + d)$, so the risk ratio can be calculated as:

$$\textbf{Risk ratio} = \frac{a/(a + b)}{c/(c + d)}$$

For example, a cohort study observed that 20 out of 50 children who regularly washed their hands with soap after defecation had at least one episode of diarrhoea during the study period, compared with 20 out of 40 children who did not. The risk ratio can be calculated as $(20 \div 50)/(20 \div 40) = 0.4 \div 0.5 = 0.80$. This is interpreted as children who practise hand washing with soap being 0.8 times as likely to have diarrhoea than those who do not practise hand washing with soap. When the relative risk is lower than one, we often subtract it from one to report the difference, so in this example we might say that those who washed hands with soap have a $1 - 0.8 = 0.2$ times, or 20%, lower risk than those who did not wash hands with soap.

Odds ratio

The **odds ratio** can also be calculated from ecological, cohort or intervention studies. It is calculated as the odds of the outcome in the exposed group divided by the odds of the outcome in the unexposed group:

$$\textbf{Odds ratio} = \frac{\textbf{Odds of outcome in exposed group}}{\textbf{Odds of outcome in unexposed group}}$$

Referring to Table 3.1, the odds of cases in the total population are calculated as $(a + c)/(b + d)$. The odds in the exposed group are a/b and the odds in the unexposed group are c/d so the odds ratio can be calculated as follows:

$$\textbf{Odds ratio} = \frac{a/b}{c/d}$$

When a fraction is divided by a fraction, it can be simplified by multiplying the top and bottom of the equation by the denominators b and d:

$$\textbf{Odds ratio} = \frac{a/b}{c/d} \times \frac{b \times d}{b \times d} = \frac{ad}{bc}$$

A variant and more frequently used version is the **odds ratio of exposure**. This is used in a case-control study because individuals are selected on the basis of their outcome status and the incidence of the outcome cannot be measured (see Chapter 9). It is calculated as the odds of exposure in individuals with the outcome divided by the odds of exposure in individuals without the outcome:

$$\text{Odds ratio of exposure} = \frac{\text{Odds of exposure in those with the outcome}}{\text{Odds of exposure in those without the outcome}}$$

Referring to Table 3.1, the odds of exposure in those with the outcome is a/c, and the odds of exposure in those without the outcome is b/d, so the odds ratio of exposure is:

$$\text{Odds ratio of exposure} = \frac{a/c}{b/d} = \frac{a/c}{b/d} \times \frac{c \times d}{c \times d} = \frac{ad}{bc}$$

As you can see, the odds ratio of exposure is mathematically the same as the odds ratio of outcome given above. The odds ratio of exposure is therefore used as an estimate of the relative risk of an outcome in case-control studies.

However, it is important not to use the terms interchangeably, as their definitions are very different. You can practise preparing 2×2 tables using the same format as Table 3.1, to work through the following examples.

One thousand mothers of newborns in a Sub-Saharan African country were asked about their level of education, of which 400 had completed primary education. After one year, there were 16 deaths among infants 'exposed' to mothers who had completed primary education and 48 deaths among 'unexposed' infants. The odds ratio of *outcome* can be calculated as $(16 \div 384)/(48 \div 552) = 0.48$. Again, as this is less than 1, we calculate the difference from 1 as $1 - 0.48 = 0.52$ and interpret it as 52% lower (than 1) odds of dying in infancy among those born to mothers who had completed primary education compared with those who had not.

In a case-control study in the same country, 100 infant deaths were identified among hospital admissions, and 100 infants who survived were selected for comparison from admissions to the same hospital. In a questionnaire conducted at admission, 20 of the mothers of infants who subsequently died reported that they had completed primary education, compared with 35 of the mothers of infants who survived. The odds ratio of *exposure* to maternal primary education can be calculated as $(20 \div 80)/(35 \div 65) = 0.250 \div 0.538 = 0.46$. This can be reported as $1 - 0.46 = 0.54$ or 54% lower odds of having a mother who had completed primary education among infants who died compared with those who survived. While we know that this is mathematically equivalent to the odds ratio of outcome, we cannot calculate the odds ratio of outcome. This is because we do not know the odds or likelihood of the outcome in the study population, having specifically selected infants for the study because they died in infancy.

Incidence rate ratio

The **incidence rate ratio** can be obtained from ecological, cohort or intervention studies. It is calculated as the incidence rate of the outcome in the exposed group divided by the incidence rate of the outcome in the unexposed group:

$$\text{Incidence rate ratio} = \frac{\text{Incidence rate of outcome in the exposed group}}{\text{Incidence rate of outcome in the unexposed group}}$$

Referring again to Table 3.1, the column for 'no outcome' would in this instance refer to the person-time at risk. The incidence rate of the outcome in the total sample population can then be calculated as $(a+c)/(b+d)$. The incidence rate in the exposed group is a/b and the incidence rate in the unexposed group is c/d. As with the odds ratio, the incidence rate ratio can be simplified as follows:

$$\textbf{Incidence rate ratio} = \frac{a/b}{c/d} = \frac{ad}{bc}$$

We use incidence rate ratio in studies where people are entering and leaving the study population or have changing levels of exposure. As an example, we might want to find out whether miners are at a higher risk of tuberculosis. We would compare the incidence rate of tuberculosis in miners (exposed group) with the incidence rate in non-miners (unexposed group). Since the miners will have worked for different lengths of time, the number of person-years at risk can be used to calculate the incidence rate in each group. If the incidence of tuberculosis in miners is 3 cases per 100 person-years and the rate for non-miners is 0.6 cases per 100 person-years, the incidence rate ratio is calculated as $3 \div 0.6 = 5$. This can be interpreted as the incidence of tuberculosis being five times as high in miners as in non-miners.

Comparability of measures of association

For common diseases (e.g. most infectious diseases), the estimates obtained may differ substantially, however, for very rare outcomes (e.g. most cancers, congenital malformations) these measures will be very similar. To demonstrate this, if we complete Table 3.1 with five cases among 5,005 exposed and 1 case among 10,001 unexposed, then we calculate:

- prevalence ratio = $(5 \div 5{,}005)/(1 \div 10{,}001) = 0.000999 \div 0.00009999 = 9.99$
- risk ratio = $(5 \div 5{,}005)/(1 \div 10{,}001) = 0.000999 \div 0.00009999 = 9.99$
- odds ratio of outcome = $(5 \div 5{,}000)/(1 \div 10{,}000) = 0.001 \div 0.0001 = 10.00$
- odds ratio of exposure = $(5 \div 1)/(5{,}000 \div 10{,}000) = 5 \div 0.5 = 10.00$
- incidence rate ratio = $(5 \div 5{,}005)/(1 \div 10{,}001) = 0.000999 \div 0.00009999 = 9.99$

The rarer the outcome, the more the denominator for the odds resembles the denominator for the risk, and the more similar are the measures of association. If the exposure were more common, then this would be even more so. For example, if there were five cases among 10,005 exposed and 1 case among 10,001 unexposed, we can calculate:

- risk ratio = $(5/10{,}005)/(1/10{,}001) = 0.00049975 \div 0.00009999 = 4.998$
- odds ratio of outcome = $(5/10{,}000)/(1/10{,}000) = 0.0005 \div 0.0001 = 5.00$

You will often see the odds ratio (of outcome) presented in a study that has measured prevalence or risk. It is used to approximate the prevalence ratio or risk ratio because of its role in complex statistical models for analysis (see Chapter 5). However, it is worth remembering that this approximation is only valid for a very rare outcome, and the odds ratio will tend to overestimate the prevalence ratio or risk ratio if the outcome is not sufficiently rare.

Activity 3.1

Investigators followed a population of 2,000 women aged over 65 years who did not have osteoporosis, over a 10-year period and measured the number of cases of osteoporosis diagnosed during that time-period. The investigators were interested in the effect of regular exercise on the development of osteoporosis. They divided the women into two groups: 1,000 women who exercised regularly (exposed) and 1,000 women who did not exercise regularly (unexposed).

During the 10-year study period, investigators recorded 800 new cases of osteoporosis, 300 in those women who exercised regularly and 500 in those who did not. The number of person-years at risk was 8,350 in the exposed group and 6,950 in the unexposed group.

1 Calculate the risk ratio, odds ratio and incidence rate ratio for the effect of regular exercise on osteoporosis in these women and provide a one-sentence interpretation for each result.
2 Contrast the findings of these measures of association, and discuss which measure is most appropriate.

Investigators then conducted another study of osteoporosis in women aged under 55 years old. They followed 1,000 women who exercised regularly and 1,000 women who did not for 10 years. They recorded 3 cases of osteoporosis in those who exercised regularly and 5 cases in those who did not. The number of person-years at risk was 9,500 in the exposed group and 9,000 in the unexposed group.

3 Again, calculate the risk ratio, odds ratio and incidence rate ratio for the effect of regular exercise on osteoporosis in these 2,000 younger women, and provide a one-sentence interpretation for each of these results.
4 Describe differences you see in the results from the two studies.

You have been introduced to several important new concepts that form the basis of epidemiology. You may find it useful to take time to digest this information before continuing with the rest of this chapter.

Measures of attributable risk

Relative measures are useful when we want to know how strongly an exposure is associated with a particular outcome, but they do not give any indication of the real impact of exposure on the incidence of outcome in a specific population. Imagine that the risk of mortality due to outcome A is six times greater in those exposed to factor A, and similarly the mortality due to outcome B is six times greater in those exposed to factor B. The incidence rate ratio is equal for both outcomes (see Table 3.2).

Table 3.2 Comparison of mortality rates for two outcomes

Epidemiological measure	Outcome A	Outcome B
Incidence rate in exposed	6 per 1,000 person-years	30 per 1,000 person-years
Incidence rate in unexposed	1 per 1,000 person-years	5 per 1,000 person-years
Incidence rate ratio	6 ÷ 1 = 6.0	30 ÷ 5 = 6.0

Source: Ilona Carneiro, modified from Bailey et al. (2005).

However, it is clear from Table 3.2 that the health impact of the exposure to factor B is greater than exposure to factor A because the underlying mortality rate is greater for outcome B than outcome A. The measure of relative risk is unable to capture this important difference, and we need to use different measures that take into account the incidence of the outcome.

Attributable risk is the excess incidence of the outcome that we can 'attribute' to the exposure, if we assume a *causal* association between the exposure and outcome. It is calculated by subtracting the underlying incidence (as a risk or a rate) of outcome in unexposed individuals from that in exposed individuals in the same population:

Attributable risk = Incidence in exposed – Incidence in unexposed

In the example above (Table 3.2), the incidence rate of outcome A that is attributable to the exposure is calculated as 6 − 1 = 5 deaths per 1,000 person-years at risk, while the incidence of outcome B that is attributable to the exposure is calculated as 30 − 5 = 25 deaths per 1,000 person-years at risk. This measure of *attributable risk* reveals the relative importance of the two exposures, based on the underlying incidence of the outcomes and is useful for comparing individual-level risks. How much worse is it for an individual in this population to be exposed to factor B than factor A? Although the relative risk of death is six times greater for exposure to either risk factor, the *actual* risk of death is five times greater (25 ÷ 5 = 5) if an individual is exposed to factor B than if they are exposed to factor A.

The **attributable fraction** is the *proportion* (fraction) of the outcome *in exposed individuals* that can be attributed to the exposure, and is calculated as:

$$\text{Attributable fraction} = \frac{\text{Incidence in exposed} - \text{Incidence in unexposed}}{\text{Incidence in exposed}}$$

or

$$\text{Attributable fraction} = \frac{\text{Attributable risk}}{\text{Incidence in exposed}}$$

In the example from Table 3.2, the attributable fraction for outcome A is $(6 - 1) \div 6 = 0.83$, i.e. 83% of deaths from outcome A can be attributed to exposure to factor A. This means that 83% of deaths from outcome A could be prevented if we were able to remove exposure to factor A completely. For outcome B, the attributable fraction is $(30 - 5) \div 30 = 0.83$, so 83% of deaths from outcome B can be attributed to exposure to factor B.

The attributable fraction is the same for both outcomes because it is related to the relative risk (risk ratio or incidence rate ratio) in the following way:

$$\textbf{Attributable fraction} = \frac{\textbf{Relative risk} - \textbf{I}}{\textbf{Relative risk}}$$

In the example from Table 3.2 this can be calculated as $(6 - 1) \div 6 = 0.83$, i.e. 83% for both outcome A and B. This is a useful approach if we do not know the actual incidence of the outcome.

For a *protective factor* where the incidence among the unexposed is greater than the incidence in the exposed, we calculate the **preventable fraction** as:

$$\textbf{Preventable fraction} = \frac{\textbf{Incidence in unexposed} - \textbf{Incidence in exposed}}{\textbf{Incidence in unexposed}}$$

This refers to the proportion of outcome incidence that can be prevented by a protective factor (e.g. genetic attribute) and can also be calculated from the relative risk:

Preventable fraction = I − Relative risk

When used to describe an intervention (e.g. a vaccine against an infectious disease), this may be referred to as the **protective efficacy** (see Chapter 10).

Population attributable risk and fraction

We may want to apply the measures of relative risk or attributable risk from an epidemiological study to a real population to enable appropriate public health planning. The **population attributable risk** (PAR) is the incidence of outcome in the population (i.e. exposed and unexposed to the risk factor) that can be attributed to the exposure of interest if we assume *causality*. It is calculated as the difference (excess risk) in incidence between the population and those individuals unexposed to the risk factor:

Population attributable risk = Incidence in population − Incidence in unexposed

For example, a study of the effect of chronic hepatitis B infection on liver cancer found the following results: the incidence rate of liver cancer was 4 per 100,000 person-years in those without chronic hepatitis B infection and 94 per 100,000 person-years in the entire population. The population attributable risk of exposure to chronic hepatitis B was calculated as $94 - 4 = 90$ per 100,000 person-years. This can be interpreted as 90 per 100,000 liver cancer cases in this study population can be attributed to chronic hepatitis B infection, and could be avoided if hepatitis B infection were to be eliminated from the population.

The **population attributable fraction** (PAF) is therefore the *proportion* (fraction) of the outcome in the *population* that is attributable to the exposure, and is calculated as:

$$\textbf{Population attributable fraction} = \frac{\textbf{Incidence in population} - \textbf{Incidence in unexposed}}{\textbf{Incidence in population}}$$

or

$$\text{Population attributable fraction } = \frac{\textbf{Population attributable risk}}{\textbf{Incidence in population}}$$

For the study of liver cancer described above, we can calculate the PAF as (94 − 4) ÷ 94 = 0.96, so 96% of liver cancer cases in the population are attributable to chronic hepatitis B infection.

The PAF can also be expressed in terms of the relative risk, as long as the proportion of the total population exposed to the risk factor ('p') is known:

$$\text{Population attributable fraction } = \frac{p \times (\textbf{Relative risk} - 1)}{p \times (\textbf{Relative risk} - 1) + 1}$$

In the example above, the researchers found the rate of liver cancer in the *study sample* to be 602 per 100,000 person-years in those with chronic hepatitis B infection and 4 per 100,000 person-years in those without hepatitis B. The prevalence of chronic hepatitis B infection in the *general population* was 15%. If the incidence rate of liver cancer in the general population had not been known, they could have calculated the incidence rate ratio as 602 ÷ 4 = 150.5. An incidence rate ratio of 150.5 is huge, but it is difficult to translate such a figure into real public health impact. The PAF calculated from the relative risk is (0.15 × (150.5 − 1)) ÷ (0.15 × (150.5 − 1) + 1) = 22.425 ÷ 23.425 = 0.96. This suggests that 96% of liver cancer cases could be eliminated if chronic hepatitis B infection could be eliminated, assuming that the association is causal. Note that there are often several risk factors for an outcome that may overlap or interact (component causes − see Chapter 1), such that reducing exposure to one risk factor may result in an increase in the *proportion* of cases due to another risk factor.

The comparative value of the attributable fraction and the population attributable fraction can be illustrated by the following hypothetical example. A study determined the risk of repetitive strain injury (RSI) to the hand in office workers to be 4 per 100 over a one-year period. Among those who used a computer keyboard for more than 5 hours a day, this risk was 10 per 100 person-years, while for those who used a computer keyboard for less than 5 hours the risk was 3 per 100 person-years. The attributable fraction identifies the proportion of RSI due to using a computer keyboard among those who use keyboards, and is calculated as (10 − 3) ÷ 10 = 0.70 or 70%. The population attributable fraction identifies the proportion of RSI due to using a computer keyboard for more than 5 hours a day among all the office workers, calculated as (4 − 3) ÷ 4 = 0.25 or 25%. In considering whether to invest in ergonomic keyboards, the employer may not consider a 25% increased risk in RSI overall to be of sufficient importance, whereas the individual would consider a 70% increase in their own risk of RSI to be considerable. This would advocate for a workstation assessment followed by a needs-based provision of ergonomic keyboards.

Activity 3.2

Between 1951 and 1971, a total of 10,000 deaths were recorded among 34,440 male British doctors (Doll and Peto 1976). Of these deaths, 441 were from lung cancer and 3,191 were from ischaemic heart disease (IHD). Doctors who smoked at least one cigarette per day during this follow-up period were classified as smokers and the rest as non-smokers. The age-adjusted annual death rates per 100,000 male doctors for lung cancer and IHD among smokers and non-smokers are given in Table 3.3. (Note that this is a comparative table, not a 2×2 table of outcome by exposure.)

Table 3.3 Cause of death and specific death rates by smoking habits of British male doctors, 1951–71

	Annual death rate per 100,000 doctors	
Cause of death	Non-smokers	Smokers
Lung cancer	10	140
Ischaemic heart disease	413	669

Source: Doll and Peto (1976).

1 Calculate an appropriate epidemiological measure to assess the strength of association between smoking and lung cancer, and smoking and IHD.
2 Based on your calculation, which of the two diseases is most strongly associated with smoking?
3 Reduction in mortality from which of the two diseases would have greater public health impact if there were a reduction in smoking? Calculate and interpret an appropriate epidemiological measure and list the assumptions you would make when estimating the impact of a reduction in smoking.
4 Assuming that the data shown in Table 3.3 are valid and that smoking causes lung cancer, how much of the mortality from lung cancer could be attributable to smoking? Assuming that smoking is one of the causes of IHD, how much of the mortality from IHD could be attributable to smoking?

Activity 3.3

A separate case-control study was conducted to investigate the risk factors for myocardial infarction. Information on smoking was collected from cases and controls. Sixty of the 400 myocardial infarction cases reported current cigarette smoking, defined as smoking within the past 3 months, compared with 40 of the 400 healthy controls.

1 Set up a 2×2 table showing the information above.
2 Calculate and interpret an appropriate measure to estimate the strength of the association between current cigarette smoking and myocardial infarction.

Activity 3.4

The incidence of tuberculosis and the mid-year population of different ethnic groups in a European country, country Z, in 2011 are given in Table 3.4.

1 Calculate the incidence rate and rate ratio for each 'exposure' group, using the European group as the reference ('unexposed') group.
2 Based on your calculations, which group is most strongly associated with tuberculosis in this study?

Table 3.4 Incidence of tuberculosis and mid-year population by ethnic group in country Z, 2011

Ethnic group	New tuberculosis cases, 2011	Mid-year population, 2011
European	2,890	69,900,000
Indian	1,900	1,790,000
Sri Lankan	400	1,650,000
Total	5,190	73,340,000

Source: Adapted from Bailey et al. (2005).

3 Explain why the number of tuberculosis cases is greater in the European group even though the incidence rate is lower than in the other two groups.

4 The incidence rate for the entire population is 7.08 per 100,000 person-years. If you assume that a targeted intervention could reduce the incidence rate in all groups to the level of that in the European group (4.13 per 100,000 person-years), what percentage of tuberculosis cases in each group would be prevented?

5 If a targeted intervention reduced the incidence rate in all groups to that of the European group, what percentage of tuberculosis cases in the whole population would be prevented?

Conclusion

You have been introduced to the relative measures (prevalence ratio, risk ratio, odds ratio and incidence rate ratio) that are used to quantify the association between an exposure and an outcome. These measures are the foundation of analytical epidemiology, and you will have the opportunity to consider them in context in subsequent chapters relating to specific study designs. You have also been introduced to measures of impact (attributable risk, attributable fraction) and population measures of impact (population attributable risk and population attributable fraction) that are needed to translate research findings into information of public health value.

References

Bailey L, Vardulaki K, Langham J and Chandramon D (2005) *Introduction to Epidemiology* 1st edn. Maidenhead: Open University Press.

Doll R and Peto R (1976) Mortality in relation to smoking: 20 years' observations on male British doctors. *British Medical Journal* 2: 1525–36.

Feedback to activities

Activity 3.1

1 To calculate the risk ratio, first calculate the incidence risk of osteoporosis in both exposed and unexposed women:

Risk in women who exercised regularly = 300 ÷ 1,000 = 0.3 per 10 years.
Risk in women who did not exercise regularly = 500 ÷ 1,000 = 0.5 per 10 years.

Then divide the incidence risk in the exposed group by the incidence risk in the unexposed group:

$$\text{Risk ratio} = \frac{0.3}{0.5} = 0.6$$

A risk ratio of 0.60 indicates that women over age 65 who exercise regularly have a 40% lower risk of developing osteoporosis than women over age 65 who do not exercise regularly, in this study population.

To calculate the odds ratio, first calculate the odds of osteoporosis in women who exercised regularly and in those who did not:

Odds in women who exercised regularly = 300 ÷ (1,000 − 300) = 300 ÷ 700 = 0.43.
Odds in women who did not exercise regularly = 500 ÷ (1,000 − 500) = 500 ÷ 500 = 1.
    Then divide the odds in the exposed group by the odds in the unexposed group:

$$\text{Odds ratio} = \frac{0.43}{1.00} = 0.43$$

An odds ratio of 0.43 indicates that women over age 65 who exercise regularly have a 57% lower odds of developing osteoporosis than women who do not exercise regularly, in this study population.
    To calculate the rate ratio, first calculate the incidence rate of osteoporosis in women who exercised regularly and in those who did not:

Incidence rate in women who exercised regularly = 300 ÷ 8,350 person-years = 0.03593 per person-year = 35.93 per 1,000 person-years. (You may have multiplied by 100 to get a rate of 3.59 per 100 person-years, which is also correct as long as the units are clearly stated, and the same units are used throughout the calculation.)
    Incidence rate in women who did not exercise regularly = 500 ÷ 6,950 person-years = 0.07194 per person-year = 71.94 per 1,000 person-years (make sure you remain consistent with the previous rate in the unit of person-years used for the denominator).
    Then divide the incidence rate in the exposed group by the incidence rate in the unexposed group:

$$\text{Rate ratio} = \frac{35.93}{71.94} = 0.50$$

A rate ratio of 0.50 indicates that women over age 65 who exercise regularly have a 50% lower rate of osteoporosis than women who do not exercise regularly, in this study population.
2 As this is a long cohort study, the rate ratio is probably the most appropriate measure as it takes into account the actual person-years at risk in the exposed and unexposed groups.
3 For the study on younger women, start by calculating the risk ratio:

Risk in younger women who exercised regularly = 3 ÷ 1,000 = 0.003 per 10 years.
Risk in women who did not exercise regularly = 5 ÷ 1,000 = 0.005 per 10 years.
Then divide the risk in the exposed group by the risk in the unexposed group:

$$\text{Risk ratio} = \frac{0.003}{0.005} = 0.60$$

A risk ratio of 0.60 indicates that women under age 55 who exercise regularly have a 40% lower risk of developing osteoporosis than women under age 55 who do not, in this study population.

For the odds ratio, first calculate the odds of osteoporosis in younger women who exercised regularly and in those who did not:

Odds in women who exercised regularly = 3 ÷ (1,000 − 3) = 3 ÷ 997 = 0.003.
Odds in women who did no regular exercise = 5 ÷ (1,000 − 5) = 5 ÷ 995 = 0.005.
Then divide the odds in the exposed group by the odds in the unexposed group:

$$\textbf{Odds ratio} \ = \ \frac{0.003}{0.005} \ = \ \textbf{0.60}$$

An odds ratio of 0.60 indicates that women under age 55 who exercise regularly have a 40% lower odds of developing osteoporosis than women under age 55 who do not, in this study population.

Calculate the rate ratio, by first calculating the incidence rate of osteoporosis in younger women who exercised regularly and in those who did not:

Rate in women who exercised regularly = 3 ÷ 9,500 person-years = 0.00032 per person-year = 0.32 per 1,000 person-years (or, perhaps more intuitively, 3.16 per 10,000 person-years).

Rate in women who did not exercise regularly = 5 ÷ 9,000 person-years = 0.00056 per person-year = 0.56 per 1,000 person-years.

Then divide the incidence rate in the exposed group by the incidence rate in the unexposed group:

$$\textbf{Rate ratio} \ = \ \frac{0.32}{0.56} \ = \ \textbf{0.57}$$

A rate ratio of 0.57 indicates that women aged under age 55 who exercise regularly have a 43% lower rate of developing osteoporosis than women under age 55 who do not, in this study population.

4 You probably noticed that in the study of women aged over 65 years, the measures of association gave somewhat different estimates for risk ratio, odds ratio, and rate ratio. This is because the outcome of interest was common. By contrast, in the study of women under 55 years, the measures of effect gave very similar estimates for risk ratio, odds ratio, and rate ratio. This is because the outcome of interest was rare.

Activity 3.2

1 An appropriate measure to assess the strength of an association in this example would be the incidence *rate ratio* because we know the incidence *rate* in each group. Rate ratio of lung cancer in smokers compared to non-smokers:

$$\textbf{Rate ratio} \ = \ \frac{140 \text{ per } 100,000}{10 \text{ per } 100,000} \ = \ \textbf{14.00}$$

Rate ratio of ischaemic heart disease (IHD) in smokers compared to non-smokers:

$$\textbf{Rate ratio} \ = \ \frac{669 \text{ per } 100,000}{413 \text{ per } 100,000} \ = \ \textbf{1.62}$$

2 A rate ratio of 14.00 for the association of smoking with lung cancer compared to a rate ratio of 1.62 for the association of smoking with IHD indicates that smoking is much more strongly associated with lung cancer than it is with IHD.

3 To assess the impact of smoking, the excess mortality attributable to smoking must be estimated. An appropriate measure to assess this is the attributable risk:

Attributable risk of smoking for lung cancer = (140 per 100,000) – (10 per 100,000) = 130 per 100,000.
Attributable risk of smoking for IHD = (669 per 100,000) – (413 per 100,000) = 256 per 100,000.

An attributable risk of smoking for lung cancer of 130 per 100,000 compared to an attributable risk of smoking for IHD of 256 per 100,000 indicates that, among smokers, a reduction in smoking would prevent far more deaths from IHD than from lung cancer. Among non-smokers, the death rate from lung cancer is fairly low (10 per 100,000), while the death rate from IHD is 413 per 100,000. The 1.62 times increase in IHD mortality associated with smoking affects a much larger number of people than the 14-fold increase in the risk of death from lung cancer. Thus, the potential public health impact of a reduction in smoking on mortality is far greater for IHD than for lung cancer. To arrive at the conclusions above, you would need to assume that smoking is causally related to lung cancer and to IHD, and that smoking is responsible for an equal proportion of the mortality from both of these diseases.

4 To assess what percentage of the risk of death from lung cancer could be attributed to smoking, you would calculate the attributable fraction. There are two ways you could calculate this:

Attributable fraction = attributable risk in smokers divided by risk in smokers:

$$\textbf{Attributable fraction} \quad = \quad \frac{\textbf{(130 per 100,000)}}{\textbf{(140 per 100,000)}} \quad = \quad \textbf{0.93}$$

Alternatively, the attributable fraction can be calculated from the relative risk of lung cancer in smokers compared to non-smokers as follows:

$$\textbf{Attributable fraction} \quad = \quad \frac{14 - 1}{14} \quad = \quad \textbf{0.93}$$

This can be interpreted as 93% of deaths from lung cancer among smokers being attributable to smoking.

Similarly, the attributable-fraction of IHD deaths among smokers is calculated as:

$$\textbf{Attributable fraction} \quad = \quad \frac{\textbf{256 per 100,000}}{\textbf{669 per 10,000}} \quad = \quad \textbf{0.38}$$

or

$$\textbf{Attributable fraction} \quad = \quad \frac{1.62 - 1}{1.62} \quad = \quad \textbf{0.38}$$

This can be interpreted as 38% of deaths from IHD among smokers being due to smoking.

Activity 3.3

1 Your table should look like Table 3.5.

Table 3.5 Odds of smoking in cases of myocardial infarction (MI) and controls

Exposure	MI (Cases)	No MI (Controls)	Total
Current smokers	60	40	100
Non-smokers	340	360	700
Total	400	400	800

Source: Natasha Howard.

2 As this is a case-control study, an appropriate measure to assess the strength of association between smoking and myocardial infarction (MI) is the odds ratio of exposure.

$$\text{Odds ratio of exposure} = \frac{60 \div 340}{40 \div 360} = \frac{60 \times 360}{40 \times 340} = 1.59$$

An odds ratio of 1.59 indicates that the odds of cigarette smoking are 1.59 times (or 59% if we calculate the difference from 1) higher in cases of MI compared to healthy controls, in this study population. *Note* it is incorrect to say that the odds of MI are 1.59 times greater in smokers than in non-smokers as we do not know the incidence, and therefore cannot calculate the odds, of MI in the study population.

Activity 3.4

1 The incidence rate and rate ratio for tuberculosis in each group is given in Table 3.6.

Table 3.6 Incidence of tuberculosis, mid-year population, incidence rate and rate ratio by ethnic group in country Z, 2011

Ethnic group	New tuberculosis cases, 2011	Mid-year population, 2011	Incidence rate per 100,000	Rate ratio
European	2,890	69,900,000	4.13	1
Indian	1,900	1,790,000	106.15	25.70
Sri Lankan	400	1,650,000	24.24	5.87
Total	5,190	73,340,000	7.08	–

Source: Adapted from Bailey et al. (2005).

2 The rate ratio is 25.70 times as high in the Indian group as in the European group and 5.87 times as high in the Sri Lankan group as in the European group. Thus, Indian ethnicity is more strongly associated with tuberculosis than are either European or Sri Lankan ethnicity.

We can also change the reference ('unexposed') to the Sri Lankan group to show that the rate ratio between Indian and Sri Lankan ethnicity is 106.15 ÷ 24.24 = 4.38.

3 The total number of tuberculosis cases is greater in the European group because the mid-year population in this group is much higher. Even though the incidence rate is

lower than in the other two groups, the European group constitutes 95% (69,900,000 ÷ 73,340,000 = 0.95) of the population.

4 Assuming that a targeted intervention has reduced the incidence rate in the Indian and Sri Lankan groups to 4.13 per 100,000, an appropriate measure to calculate the proportion of tuberculosis cases in the Indian group prevented by the intervention would be the preventable fraction. The current rate is taken as the rate in those unexposed to the intervention and the reduced rate is taken as the rate in those exposed to the intervention:

$$\frac{\textbf{Rate in unexposed} - \textbf{Rate in exposed}}{\textbf{Rate in unexposed}} = \frac{106.15 - 4.13}{106.15} = 0.96$$

A preventable fraction of 0.96 or 96% means that if the incidence rate in the Indian group were reduced to the level of the European group, then 96% of tuberculosis cases in the Indian population must have been prevented by the intervention. Similarly for the Sri Lankan group, the preventable fraction is calculated as:

$$\frac{\textbf{Rate in unexposed} - \textbf{Rate in exposed}}{\textbf{Rate in unexposed}} = \frac{24.24 - 4.13}{24.24} = 0.83$$

This means that the intervention would prevent 0.83 or 83% of tuberculosis cases in the Sri Lankan population.

5 Assuming the incidence rate in Indian and Sri Lankan groups is reduced to 4.13 per 100,000, an appropriate measure of the percentage reduction of tuberculosis cases in the whole population attributable to the intervention, is the population attributable fraction:

$$\frac{\textbf{Population rate} - \textbf{Reduced rate}}{\textbf{Population rate}} = \frac{7.08 - 4.13}{7.08} = 0.42$$

A population attributable fraction of 0.42 or 42% means that if the incidence rate in all groups were reduced to the level of the European group, then 42% of tuberculosis cases would be prevented by the intervention in the whole population.

Interpreting associations 4

Overview

Epidemiological measures of association between an exposure and outcome cannot be used to infer causality unless alternative explanations have been excluded. In this chapter you will learn about alternative explanations for an apparent association: chance, bias and confounding. The role of these effects needs to be considered when designing a study, and assessed whenever an association is found. To finally infer causality, it is necessary to build up supportive evidence, for example by using the Bradford-Hill list of considerations for causality.

Learning objectives

When you have completed this chapter you should be able to:

- distinguish between chance, bias and confounding as alternative explanations for an apparent association between an exposure and an outcome
- explain the concept of chance in relation to measures of frequency and measures of association
- describe how different types of selection bias and information bias may distort measures of association
- identify confounding factors and be aware of how to control for their effects in the analysis
- specify methods for avoiding chance, bias and confounding in study design
- distinguish between statistical association and causality
- list the nine considerations for supporting causality.

Critical appraisal

The ultimate aim of analytical epidemiology is to show whether a measured association between an exposure and outcome is causal, providing a target for subsequent public health interventions. In the previous chapter, you learned about relative measures of association, and the need to assume causality in order to estimate the impact of an exposure. However, before we can infer causality, it is necessary to critically appraise the evidence and exclude other possible reasons for a measured association. The three main alternative explanations for an observed epidemiological association are **chance**, **bias** and **confounding**. Once these have been excluded, it is then necessary to consider whether there is sufficient evidence that an association is likely to be causal.

Chance and statistical probability

In both descriptive and analytical studies, we make inferences about a population from a sample of individuals. It is usually not feasible to measure the outcome and/or exposure in every member of a given population or subgroup. There is, therefore, a *chance* that if the sample were repeated with different individuals, the result would be different. For example, consider that we want to know the number of children who have received three doses of diptheria-tetanus-pertussis (DTP3) vaccine, as a marker of access to routine child health interventions for a region of country X. If we question the mothers of 10 infants at random, and then repeat this several times for different infants, we would most likely get a different prevalence of DTP3 coverage each time. One way to reduce the variability in our results would be to increase the number of infants we sampled. As this **sample size** increases, the sample becomes more representative of the population of interest, and this is therefore the main way to reduce the role of chance in an epidemiological study.

Statistical analysis of results can then be used to assess how representative a sample was of the population of interest, and this is described by two measures: the *P*-value and the confidence interval. Both of these are based on sampling variation and the fact that many variables show a normal distribution, also known as a bell-shaped curve (as shown in Figure 4.1). Consider a DTP3 survey of 100 infants in a population where the 'true' coverage is 75%. Figure 4.1 shows the distribution of prevalence that we might see if we repeated the sample 100 times. We would most frequently measure values close to the true population prevalence and less frequently measure values higher or lower than this. The height and width of the curve will vary according to the amount of variation in the prevalence of DTP3 in the population.

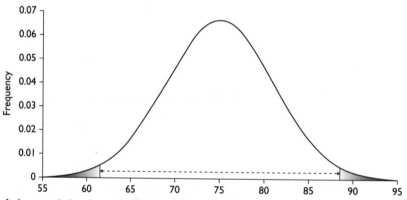

Figure 4.1 A normal distribution or 'bell-shaped' curve, illustrating the 95% confidence interval as a dashed line

Source: Ilona Carneiro.

The **P-value** is the probability that an observed value or association from a sample occurred by chance alone, and that it does *not* exist in the population from which the sample was selected. A *P*-value of less than or equal to 0.05 means that there is a 5% or 1 in 20 chance that the sample result does not represent the reality. This is generally considered low enough to imply that the result is not due to chance. However, this should be used as a guide and not as fixed threshold for reporting the **statistical significance**. For example, in a study of diarrhoea in children given iron supplementation compared with a placebo, if the incidence rate ratio = 1.20, P = 0.04, we would interpret this as *borderline* statistically significant evidence of an increased risk, requiring further investigation.

The **confidence interval** is the range of values, estimated from a sample, within which the 'true' population value is likely to be found. In Figure 4.1, if the area under the curve represents the results of 100 samples of DTP3 coverage, then the unshaded area represents the results of 95 of these samples. The values at either end of this unshaded area are known as the limits of the confidence interval. In this example, we can say that we have 95% confidence that the DTP3 coverage in the population is between 61–89%. This means that if we were to repeat the random sample 100 times, 95 times out of 100 we would obtain a result that lies within this interval. The wider the confidence interval is, the less precision we have about the true value (i.e. the more possible numbers that could be the true value).

For a measure of association (prevalence ratio, odds ratio, risk ratio, rate ratio) where the value 1.0 represents no association, if the 95% confidence interval (CI) includes 1.0, we can say that the association is not significant at the 5% level (i.e. the P-value will be greater than 0.05). For example, if the risk ratio = 1.10 (95% CI: 0.90, 1.20), this suggests that it is not significantly different from 1.0 and there is no significant association between the exposure and outcome. If the entire range of the 95% CI had been greater than 1.0, we could be more confident that there was truly an increased risk of the outcome among exposed individuals.

Bias

Bias is a systematic (i.e. non-random) error that leads to an incorrect measure of association. Sample size does not affect bias, and statistical methods cannot be used to adjust for bias; it must, therefore, be avoided through appropriate study design. The **random selection** of study participants or **random allocation** of individuals to comparison groups aims to reduce systematic bias, but does not completely prevent it. Bias can be categorized as either selection bias or information bias.

Selection bias

Selection bias occurs when there is a systematic difference between the characteristics of individuals sampled and the population from which the sample is taken, or a systematic difference between the comparison groups within the study population. For example, people who volunteer to participate in a study are 'self-selected' and are likely to differ from the general population in terms of health awareness, education and other factors that may also affect the outcome of interest. Selection bias is most important in case-control studies where cases and controls should only differ on the outcome and exposure of interest. Several factors may affect whether selection bias occurs:

1 The definition of the study population or comparison group. For example, in an **occupational cohort** study where comparison is made with the general population, the overall health of the occupational cohort will usually be better than the general

population, which includes individuals who are not well enough to work. This is known as the 'healthy worker effect', and can be reduced by selecting for comparison other workers without the exposure of interest.

2 The inclusion and exclusion criteria. For example, in a study of access to routine healthcare using household lists drawn up by village elders, recent migrants or marginalized groups may be excluded from the study.

3 The rate of loss to follow-up. For example, if individuals in an intervention study receiving an active intervention are more likely to continue attending follow-up clinics than those receiving a placebo, our detection of cases will be different between the two groups. If more cases are detected in intervention than control individuals we may wrongly conclude that the intervention has failed.

Information bias

Information bias occurs when there is a systematic difference between comparison groups in the way that data are collected, and can be introduced by those measuring the outcome (observer bias), the study participants (responder bias), or measurement tools, such as weighing scales or questionnaires (measurement bias). Information bias may result in the misclassification of exposure or disease status in a non-differential (random) or differential (non-random) way.

Non-differential misclassification occurs when both comparison groups (exposed and unexposed; cases and controls) are equally likely to be misclassified. It is therefore independent of exposure or outcome status, and will not bias the direction of any observed association between exposure and outcome. However, it causes the comparison groups to appear more similar than they actually are, and may lead to an *underestimation of the strength of the association*. Always consider the potential role of non-differential misclassification when interpreting a study that appears to show no statistically significant association between the exposure and outcome.

Consider a case-control study of the association of oral contraceptive use with ovarian cancer, using 20 years of clinic records to determine exposure. It is unlikely that all records of oral contraceptive use over the previous 20 years from a family planning clinic will be traceable. The loss of records would probably be distributed equally among the cases and the controls, since record keeping in family planning clinics is independent of the risk of developing cancer. However, if the investigators decided to classify all women without a record as unexposed to contraceptives, then the odds of exposure would be underestimated in both cases and controls. This would lead to underestimation of the effect of contraceptives on ovarian cancer.

Differential misclassification occurs when classification of the exposure is dependent on the outcome or vice versa, and is generally due to observer or responder bias. It can lead to the over- or underestimation of a measure of association, and may also lead to false associations.

For example, in an intervention study of the effect of promoting regular exercise among the elderly on blood pressure, a visiting health worker may under-estimate the blood pressure of those known to be receiving the intervention, or over-estimate the blood pressure of those known to not be receiving the intervention.

Observer bias refers to misclassification caused by the observer's knowledge of the comparison group. This may not be deliberate, or very large, but if it is systematically high or low, it can affect the study outcome. It may take the form of tending to 'round up' measures for one group and 'round down' measures for the other group. To reduce the effect of observer bias, the exposure status (or outcome status in a case-control study) should be concealed from the person measuring the outcome or exposure – this is known as **blinding**.

Responder bias refers to systematic differences in the information provided by a study participant, and may take the form of recall or reporting bias. For example, in a case-control study of lung cancer and exposure to secondary smoke, cases may be more likely to remember their historical experience of secondary smoke (recall bias) if they are aware of the association between smoking and cancer, overestimating the association. Similarly, in a study of sexual behaviour and prevalence of sexually transmitted infections (STIs), individuals with a higher number of sexual partners and therefore at higher risk of STIs, may also be more likely to under-report their number of partners due to social stigma (reporting bias), resulting in an under-estimate of the association.

Responder bias is reduced by 'blinding' the participants, i.e. concealing the exposure from them. This may be done by using a **placebo** in intervention trials or concealing the hypothesis under investigation in other studies. For example, investigators may ask about a wide variety of exposures rather than focusing only on the exposure of interest. They may also ask a question in several different ways to ensure consistency of responses. Recall bias can be reduced by using objective records (e.g. vaccination cards) or shortening the recall period (e.g. asking 'did you eat dairy products yesterday?' rather than within the last week).

Confounding

Confounding occurs when an apparent association between an exposure and an outcome is actually the result of another factor (**confounder**). A confounding factor must be *independently* associated with both the exposure and the outcome, and must not be on the **causal pathway** between the two (i.e. where the exposure causes an intermediary factor, which then causes the outcome). Figure 4.2 illustrates the relationship between an exposure, outcome and confounder. For example, an apparent association between occupation and lung cancer could be the result of the occupational cohort being more likely to smoke (or smokers being more likely to choose a particular occupation) and therefore at increased risk of lung cancer. A confounder does not need to cause the outcome or wholly explain the relationship between the exposure and outcome. Age and socio-economic status are two common confounders.

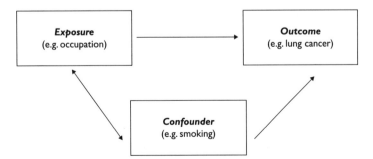

Figure 4.2 The relationship between an exposure, outcome and confounder

Source: Ilona Carneiro, modified from LSHTM lecture notes.

If the third factor is on the causal pathway between the exposure and outcome, it is not a confounder. For example, coronary heart disease is associated with high blood cholesterol, and blood cholesterol is a direct result of diet. Blood cholesterol does not provide an *alternative explanation* for the relationship between diet and coronary heart disease, but is an intermediary between them, and is therefore not a confounder.

There are three ways to avoid confounding effects when designing a study:

1 **Randomization** involves the random allocation of individuals to the exposure and control groups, such that each study participant has an equal chance of being exposed or unexposed. If the sample size is sufficiently large, this method ensures the equal distribution between exposure groups of known and *unknown* confounders. This is the best method to avoid confounding, but can only be used in intervention studies.
2 **Restriction** limits the study to people who are similar in relation to the confounder. For example, if sex is known to be a confounder, the study may only include men. However, this means that the results of the study cannot then be extrapolated to women.
3 **Matching** selects the two comparison groups to have the same distribution of potential confounders, and is generally only used in case-control studies. At an individual level it is known as 'pair matching'. For example, when looking at the effect of hygiene practices on the risk of diarrhoea, a community control of the same age is identified for each diarrhoea case. At a group level it is called 'frequency matching'. For example, when looking at exposure to smoking, female cases of lung cancer may be matched to female hospital controls and male cases matched to male controls.

There are two ways to control for confounding in the analysis, if data on confounders have been measured:

1 **Stratification** is an extension of frequency matching as it measures the association between exposure and outcome separately for each category (stratum) of a confounder. For example, in a study of the association between long-term cannabis use and cognitive function, the measure of association should be calculated separately for each age group, as age is likely to be associated with amount of cannabis exposure and independently with cognitive function. The results can then be combined to obtain a measure of association that has been *adjusted* for the effects of the confounder. Always try to limit the number of strata in the analysis, as the sample size of each stratum will be reduced, increasing the role of chance.
2 **Statistical modelling** allows us to adjust simultaneously for several confounders using methods such as multivariable **regression** analyses (see Chapter 5).

Our ability to control for confounding will depend on the accuracy with which the confounders have been measured. Non-differential (random) misclassification of a confounder would underestimate the effect of that confounder, reducing our ability to control for it. This is known as **residual confounding** and it *biases* the association between the exposure and outcome in the same direction as the confounding.

For example, a case-control study (Becher 1992) found that laryngeal cancer was associated with a four times greater odds of regular alcohol consumption (Odds Ratio = 4.22). After adjusting for the confounding effect of smoking (i.e. comparing smokers to non-smokers), this was reduced slightly to give an OR of 4.02. However, after adjusting for the average number of cigarettes smoked per day, which is more precise, the OR was 3.07. This shows that using two categories of smoking resulted in residual confounding, because it was not a sufficiently accurate measure of exposure to smoking to adjust for the confounding effect.

Activity 4.1

In each of the following examples, there is an alternative explanation for the association between the exposure and the outcome. For each example, identify the alternative explanation (bias, confounding, or chance) and why you think it occurred (imagine you are explaining your reasons to a colleague).

1 In a study of risk factors for infant mortality, the investigators find that infant mortality is significantly lower in households where the father wears a watch. The investigators therefore conclude that if watches were given to fathers, infant mortality would fall.
2 Four people want to give up smoking. At random, two of them are given garlic pills to help them stop, and two are not. The two who take garlic pills succeed in giving up smoking. The other two do not. The investigators conclude that garlic pills help people give up smoking. However, a significance test shows that $P = 0.3$.
3 In a case-control study to examine risk factors for lung cancer, cases are people admitted to hospital with lung cancer, and controls are people admitted to the same hospital with emphysema (a chronic lung disease for which smoking is a risk factor). The study finds no association between smoking and lung cancer.
4 A case-control study of Down's syndrome found that fewer mothers of cases smoked during pregnancy than didn't. After adjusting for maternal age (<35 years, ≥35 years) the effect was still negative, but not statistically significant. After adjusting for exact year of maternal age there was no association (odds ratio = 1.00).

Inferring causality

A statistically significant association between an exposure and an outcome is not sufficient to imply causality. Once alternative explanations for an observed association have been discounted or adjusted for, we must then consider whether the association is likely to be causal.

For example, in a *baseline* survey of 10,000 children, of whom half were subsequently randomized to receive an intervention, the mean haemoglobin concentration was significantly different at 11.7 compared with 11.9 g/dl. The groups are very large, have been randomized, and no interventions have yet been applied. There is therefore no explanation for any association between the randomization group and the mean haemoglobin. In addition, the magnitude of difference is very small, and it is only statistically significant as a result of the fine grading of the measurement, low variability in between children and the large sample size. We therefore have to apply our judgement as to whether a statistically significant result has epidemiological importance, or whether there is a logical basis for an observed association.

Sir Austin Bradford Hill (1965) listed nine considerations, none of which are essential, that are used in epidemiology to build-up evidence for a causal relationship:

1 *Strength*: the stronger the association between the exposure and outcome, the less likely that the relationship is due to some other factor. For example, a ten times greater odds of laryngeal cancer among heavy alcohol drinkers decreases the likelihood that the relationship is wholly confounded by some other factor. A confounder would have to be much more frequent among heavy drinkers than non-drinkers. This criterion does not imply that an association of small magnitude cannot be causal, but in such cases it is more difficult to exclude alternative explanations.

2 *Consistency*: is the repeatability of the result. If the same association has been observed from various studies and in different geographic settings, it suggests that the association is real. For example, the assessment of a cause–effect relationship between cigarette smoking and coronary heart disease has been enhanced by the fact that similar results have been obtained by a number of cohort and case-control studies conducted over 30 years in different populations.

3 *Temporality*: while it may seem obvious that the exposure *must* be present or have occurred prior to the outcome, this can be more complex to ascertain for outcomes of slow development. For example, does a particular diet lead to a digestive disorder, or do the symptoms of the disorder affect the sufferer's diet? Temporality is also not easy to establish in cross-sectional or case-control studies, where the exposure and outcome are measured simultaneously. In such cases an apparent risk factor may actually be a consequence of the outcome, this is known as **reverse causality**.

4 *Dose–response*: where there is an increased risk of outcome with increased exposure. For example, increased risk of lung cancer among heavy smokers compared with moderate smokers, and increased risk among moderate smokers compared with light smokers. However, a dose–response relationship alone does not confirm causality and the absence of a dose–response relationship does not rule out causality.

5 *Plausibility*: the existence of a reasonable biological mechanism for the cause and effect lends weight to the association, but depends on the existing knowledge. For example, a causal relationship between the moderate consumption of alcohol and decreased risk of coronary heart disease is enhanced by the fact that alcohol is known to increase the level of high-density lipoprotein, which is associated with a decreased risk of coronary heart disease. However, the lack of a known or postulated mechanism does not necessarily rule out a cause–effect relationship. For example, John Snow hypothesized that water was the source of cholera epidemics in London long before the identification of *Vibrio cholera* (see Chapter 1).

6 *Reversibility*: relates to whether an intervention to remove or reduce the exposure results in the elimination or reduction of the outcome. For example, vitamin D deficiency is associated with muscle weakness, and older people are prone to develop vitamin D deficiency. However, it is difficult to infer a causal association between vitamin D deficiency and muscle weakness in the elderly. Other conditions may also cause weakness or tiredness, preventing elderly people from going outside and being exposed to sunlight (a source of vitamin D), and thus confounding the association. Randomized intervention trials of vitamin D supplementation in the elderly have been shown to improve muscle strength and function, indicating causality (Janssen et al. 2002).

7 *Coherence*: refers to a logical consistency with other information. For example, the simultaneous increase in smoking habits and incidence of lung cancer over a period of time would support a causal link, as would isolation from cigarette smoke of factors that caused cancer in laboratory animals (Hill 1965).

8 *Analogy*: similarity with other established cause–effect relationships helps to support the argument for causality. For example, previous experience with the effects of thalidomide or rubella infection in pregnancy would lend support for a causal effect of another drug or viral infection in pregnancy with similar, but weaker, evidence.
9 *Specificity*: this relates to the relationship being specific to the outcome of interest. For example, in a study of the effect of bicycle helmets, if we saw a reduction only in head injuries and not to other parts of the body, it would strengthen the inference of a protective effect of the helmet, and reduce the likelihood that the association was confounded by factors such as helmet-wearers being more careful riders (Weiss 2002). However, many outcomes are the result of more than one exposure (see Chapter 1 on component causes). For example, smoking is a cause of coronary heart disease, however, high cholesterol is also a cause of coronary heart disease, and smoking is also a cause of lung cancer and other illnesses.

Activity 4.2

A randomized, clinical intervention trial compared the effect of miltefosine, the first oral drug for the treatment of zoonotic cutaneous leishmaniasis caused by *Leishmania major*, with standard meglumine antimoniate treatment in northeastern Iran. The outcome of interest was clinical recovery (cure) measured three months post treatment. At this time point, 26 of 32 patients receiving oral miltefosine were cured and 20 of 31 patients receiving intramuscular meglumine antimoniate were cured. No relapses were observed at six-month follow-up and both regimens were well tolerated. Investigators compared treatment results in intervention (miltefosine) and control (meglumine) groups.

1 Identify, calculate and interpret a ratio to compare treatment results after three months, using the control group as baseline. What does this tell you?
The investigators calculated a 95% confidence interval (95%CI) of 0.62 – 1.33 and P-value of 0.09 for this association measure.
2 Interpret the 95% CI and P-value shown for this study. What do these tell you?
3 How might you reduce the role of chance in this study?

Activity 4.3

A case-control study was conducted to assess the association between maternal depression and infant nutritional status in a peri-urban district of Liberia. Cases were 82 undernourished infants (low weight-for-age) recruited at the local clinic while attending for measles immunization. Controls were 82 infants (normal weight-for-age) recruited during a measles campaign in the local community and matched with cases by age and gender. Some 122 of the mothers provided informed consent and were screened for depression using a standard assessment tool.

1 Might selection of controls introduce bias into this study, and if so how?
2 Might lack of consent by some mothers introduce bias into this study, and if so how?
3 How might potential bias be reduced in this study?

Activity 4.4

A cross-sectional study was carried out to assess the association between a school-based health promotion package with adolescent use of health services in District Y of northern Ghana. The investigators were interested in exposure to school-based health promotion activities. Participants were selected randomly from 'exposed' students attending the ten schools in which the health promotion package had been implemented for the previous two years, and 'unexposed' students attending ten schools that had not implemented the package. The outcome of interest was the prevalence of self-reported attendance at health services in the previous year measured through a survey undertaken at the schools.

1 Could measurement of exposure introduce bias into this study? Give reasons for your answer.
2 Could measurement of the study outcome introduce bias into this study? Give reasons for your answer.
3 How might you reduce potential information bias in this study?

Activity 4.5

An intervention study in women of different ages showed a strong association between intense exercise and reduced risk of osteoporosis.

1 Define the concept of confounding in the context of this study.
2 Describe how this study finding could be the result of confounding.
3 How could you address potential confounding in this study?

Conclusion

You should now appreciate that epidemiological associations need to be interpreted with caution. An apparent association could be the result of chance, bias or confounding, which may be avoided by appropriate study design or adjusted for in analysis. You have been introduced to several criteria that may support causal inference in an epidemiological association. Alternative explanations and evidence for causality need to be considered when designing and undertaking an epidemiological investigation, and when interpreting the results of epidemiological studies.

References

Becher H (1992) The concept of residual confounding in regression models and some applications. *Statistics in Medicine* 11: 1747–58.
Hill A B (1965) The environment and disease: association or causation? *Proceedings of the Royal Society of Medicine* 58: 295–300.
Janssen HC, Samson MM and Verhaar HJ (2002) Vitamin D deficiency, muscle function, and falls in elderly people. *American Journal of Clinical Nutrition* 75: 611–5.
Weiss NS (2002) Can the 'specificity' of an association be rehabilitated as a basis for supporting a causal hypothesis? *Epidemiology* 13: 6–8.

Feedback to activities

Activity 4.1

1 This is an example of *confounding*. The exposure of interest is wearing a watch, which is associated with socio-economic group. Low socio-economic group is a risk factor for infant mortality. Therefore, the apparent association between wearing a watch and lower infant mortality is probably due to confounding by socio-economic group. Socio-economic group (the confounder) is an alternative explanation for the apparent association between wearing a watch (the exposure of interest) and infant mortality (the outcome).

2 In this example the result was due to *chance* or random error. This study shows an apparent association between taking garlic pills and giving up smoking, but the number of subjects is very small, and the P-value is 0.30, meaning that there is a 30% chance that this association might be seen with this sample size even if it was not real. A much larger sample size would be needed to determine if there was a real association between taking garlic pills and giving up smoking.

3 The study has been poorly designed and has resulted in *selection bias*. The controls have emphysema, which has an increased risk with smoking tobacco, suggesting that this group is more likely to smoke tobacco than the overall population that the cases came from. A more appropriate control group would be hospital admissions for an outcome that is unrelated to exposure to tobacco smoke, such that the prevalence of smoking among the controls would be the same as among the population that produced the cases.

4 This is an example of confounding – more precisely *residual confounding*. The apparent protective effect of smoking in pregnancy on Down's syndrome was confounded by maternal age. When the investigators adjusted for crude categories of maternal age, it had some effect on the odds ratio of exposure, but after they adjusted for actual maternal age there was a greater effect. Adjustment by age categories did not completely remove the effect of confounding because it was not an adequate measure of how the confounder was working.

   (It has been shown that the risk of Down's syndrome increases with maternal age. The proportion of smoking during pregnancy must have been associated with maternal age, for age to confound the association between smoking and Down's syndrome. In fact, the proportion of smoking must have shown a constant (linear) decrease with age for the continuous maternal age variable to have a greater effect on the association than the binomial categories of maternal age.)

Activity 4.2

1 The outcome is 'risk of recovery', i.e. how many people changed their infection status during a fixed time-period, therefore, an appropriate measure of association would be the risk ratio.

   The 'risk of recovery' among the intervention group was $26 \div 32 = 0.81$ or 81%. The risk of recovery among the control group was $20 \div 31 = 0.65$ or 65%. Therefore the risk ratio = $0.81 \div 0.65 = 1.25$.

   A risk ratio of 1.25 indicates that those receiving miltefosine have a 25% higher likelihood of having achieved a cure at three months than do those receiving standard meglumine treatment in this study. However, this does not tell you whether this difference is real or due to chance.

2 Evaluating the role of chance in study findings requires two related statistical assessments: (a) calculating a P-value to test the study hypothesis and determine the likelihood that sampling variability could explain study results; and (b) estimating the 95% confidence interval (CI) to indicate the range within which the true result is likely to be.

A P-value of 0.09 is relatively high, indicating a 9% probability that the study result of 1.25 may be due to chance. A 95% CI of (0.62 − 1.33) indicates that you can be 95% confident that the true risk ratio in this study population is between 0.62 and 1.33. Because this CI includes '1.00', you know that the P-value is greater than 0.05 and that the measure of association is not significant at the 5% level. The confidence interval is relatively wide, so you would not be confident of extrapolating the observed RR estimate of 1.26 to the whole population.

3 Statistical significance and confidence intervals help to evaluate the role of chance as an alternative explanation of an observed association. The most common way of reducing the role of chance is to increase sample size, which increases the magnitude of the P-value. This study sample is only 63 participants so a larger sample size might provide a more robust estimate.

Activity 4.3

1 Yes, selection of controls might introduce *selection bias* in this study. Controls were selected from the community while cases were selected from the clinic. Thus, controls may in some way be different from cases, for example in access to healthcare. This type of bias cannot be corrected through statistical techniques at the analysis stage.

2 Yes, lack of consent may cause *selection bias* (more specifically non-responder bias) in this study. There were 164 infants (82 cases and 82 controls), but only 122 mothers (122 ÷ 164 = 0.74 or 74%) agreed to be assessed for depression. A non-participant rate of 26% (100 − 74 = 26) is high, and these mothers may have been different from those participating in many ways. Additionally, we have no information about how the percentage of non-participating mothers was distributed among cases and controls and so do not know if this differed systematically between the cases and controls.

3 To reduce potential selection bias, controls could have been selected from non-malnourished infants attending for measles vaccination in the clinic.

Reducing the number of non-responders would be more challenging, but might be done through community information meetings and discussion of the aims and benefits of the research.

Activity 4.4

1 Yes, measurement of exposure to the health promotion package could cause bias in this study. We do not know what the promotion activities consisted of or whether there could be overlap ('**contamination**') between schools attended by participants categorized as 'exposed' and schools attended by participants categorized as 'unexposed'. For example, we do not know how far apart health promotion and non-promotion schools were from each other. We also do not know if there were other activities to promote health service attendance in the communities from which the 'non-exposed' students were selected. The effect of such a bias would most likely *reduce the association* between outcome and exposure.

2 Yes. Outcomes were measured through self-reporting, so information bias may have been introduced in the form of observer or reporting bias. If 'exposed' students had

been sensitized to the importance of attending health services, they might be more likely to report having attended in the past year. Additionally, one year is a long recall period and both 'exposed' and 'non-exposed' participants might not remember correctly whether they had attended services. Interviewers would be aware of participants' status as 'exposed' and 'non-exposed' as this varied by school. There is therefore a possibility that, if the interviewers were aware of the study outcome of interest, they might be more likely to record an 'exposed' participant as having attended health services.

3 Potential recall or observer bias could both be reduced through objective outcome measurement (e.g. checking health centre records). Self-reporting is subjective by nature and is therefore more prone to bias.

Activity 4.5

1 The presence of confounding would mean that the observed association between exposure (intense exercise) and outcome (reduced osteoporosis risk) is due totally or in part to the effects of another variable or variables. Such a variable must be associated with intense exercise and independently of this also be associated with osteoporosis.

2 In this study, age could act as a confounder, providing an alternative explanation for the observed association between heavy exercise and osteoporosis risk. Young women, as a group, tend to exercise more heavily. Additionally, and independently, younger women have a lower risk of osteoporosis. Note that this alternative association does not need to be causal – increased age does not necessarily cause osteoporosis.

3 The three common ways of controlling for confounding at the design stage are randomization, restriction and matching. Confounding can be addressed at the analysis stage by statistical techniques such as stratified and multivariate analyses if data on potential confounders have been collected.

SECTION 2

Epidemiological research studies

Study design and handling data   5

Overview

An epidemiological investigation starts with identifying the association of interest and choosing an appropriate study design. Then investigators employ methods to reduce the role of chance, bias and confounding, and collect data in a way that will maximize its utility. In this chapter you will learn about choosing an appropriate study design and issues of developing a protocol and data management that are common to the different epidemiological study designs. Design-specific topics will be covered in subsequent chapters.

Learning objectives

When you have completed this chapter you should be able to:

- recognize the principal study designs and select an appropriate design for a specific situation
- outline the steps for developing a study protocol, e.g. sample size calculation, sampling of subjects, design of data collection tools
- explain the need for unique identifiers and relational databases
- define both quantitative (binomial, categorical, continuous) and qualitative data types
- describe the basic approaches to analysing epidemiological data.

Choice of study design

In Chapter 1 you were introduced to descriptive and analytical sources of epidemiological data. Descriptive data provide information on the *frequency* of an *outcome* or level of *exposure*, but do not analyse an association between the outcome and exposure. Analytical studies measure the *association* between an exposure and outcome, with the aim of inferring causality.

Descriptive data may come from routinely collected data sources or epidemiological studies, and are used to identify health issues for further study. For example, a fifteen-fold increase was seen in the number of lung-cancer deaths in England and Wales between 1922 and 1947, prompting investigation of the cause of this change (Doll and Hill 1950). Routinely collected data include population censuses and population health surveys (described further in Chapter 6), vital registration systems, outcome registries and health facility data (described further in Chapter 12). Descriptive epidemiological studies may be undertaken to assess whether the burden of an outcome is of public health importance, or as part of a situational analysis for subsequent epidemiological investigation. Descriptive studies may use cross-sectional surveys or longitudinal follow-up of a cohort, and the methodological issues are the same as for analytical forms of these study designs.

There are five main types of analytical study:

1 Ecological studies compare the frequency of outcome and exposure at a *population-level*. They may use cross-sectional or cohort methods to identify epidemiological associations that then require further investigation to infer causality. Using the lung-cancer example above, mortality rates differed between urban and rural populations, lending support to the hypothesis that the risk factor may be atmospheric pollution.

2 Cross-sectional studies compare the *prevalence* of outcome with exposure status at one time-point, from a random sample of individuals. These are rapid and less costly than other studies, and may be best for common or chronic outcomes. The simultaneous collection of outcome and exposure data makes it difficult to infer causality, and these studies are often used to provide preliminary evidence of an individual-level association, e.g. population surveys of obesity and reported dietary habits.

3 Cohort studies compare the *incidence* of outcome in individuals with recorded differences in exposure. These require a well-defined population and are usually time-consuming, costly and logistically more difficult than other study designs. However, they are ideal for inferring causality, as the exposure is recorded prior to the outcome. For example, a large cohort of men working at several oil refineries, could be followed up over several years to assess whether this occupation was associated with the incidence of various causes of death.

4 Case-control studies select individuals on the basis of their outcome status and analyse whether they differ in relation to previous exposure, making them prone to selection and information bias. These are best for studying rare outcomes, or for outbreak investigations, where it would not be practical to follow-up individuals over a long period of time. Early case-control studies of AIDS (acquired immunodeficiency syndrome) identified risk groups and risk factors, resulting in the restriction of high-risk blood donors and promotion of safer behaviours even before identification of the HIV (human immunodeficiency) virus (Schulz and Grimes 2002).

5 Intervention studies allocate a protective exposure, and compare outcomes between those exposed and unexposed. These are the gold standard for inferring causality but can only be used for protective exposures, which include the removal of exposure to a risk factor. Intervention studies may combine several study designs. For example, study of a malaria control intervention may start with a baseline descriptive study, followed by a cohort study to analyse the effect on malaria incidence, and end with a cross-sectional study to analyse the effect on malaria and anaemia prevalence.

The choice of analytical design will depend on existing information about the association of interest, expected frequency of the outcome, and logistical constraints such as time, budget and personnel. Each analytical design also has different strengths and weaknesses in relation to bias and confounding (see Table 5.1).

Table 5.1 Key features, advantages and disadvantages of main epidemiological study designs

Study design	Key features	Advantages	Disadvantages
Ecological	• Population-based • Prevalent or incident cases	+ Relatively easy to collect data (routine) + Rapid + Relatively inexpensive	− Cannot show causality − High probability of confounding
Cross-sectional	• Outcome and exposure measured simultaneously • Prevalent cases • Measures association as prevalence ratio (or odds ratio if outcome is rare)	+ Relatively easy to collect data + Rapid	− Difficult to know if exposure preceded outcome (problems of information bias) − Medium probability of selection bias − Medium probability of confounding
Cohort	• Exposure determined before cases detected • Incident cases • Measure association as risk ratio, odds ratio or rate ratio	+ Low probability of selection bias + Low probability of recall bias + Low probability of confounding	− Medium to high probability of loss-to-follow-up (dependent on length of study) − Logistically more difficult − More expensive
Case control	• Participants selected by outcome with exposure determined subsequently • No measure of outcome frequency • Measures association as odds ratio of exposure	+ Low probability of loss-to-follow-up + Can be rapid	− High probability of selection bias − High probability of information bias − Medium probability of confounding
Intervention (Randomized)	• Protective measure applied or risk factor removed from one group • Prevalent or incident cases • Measures association as preventable fraction	+ Low probability of selection bias + Low probability of information bias + Very low probability of confounding	− Medium probability of loss-to-follow-up − More complex − More expensive

Source: Ilona Carneiro.

Activity 5.1

For each of the following examples identify the study design used and list the possible measures of association that could be calculated:

1 Comparison of 50 people with brain cancer and 100 people without brain cancer to identify the relative risk of brain cancer in those regularly using a mobile phone.
2 A study of 10,000 people followed up during a ten-year period to identify the risk factors for heart disease.
3 A comparison of the prevalence of anaemia (haemoglobin < 8 g/dl) at eight months gestation among women using an insecticide-treated mosquito net in pregnancy, compared with women using an untreated mosquito net in pregnancy.
4 Comparison of national infant mortality rates by gross domestic product.
5 A study of the number of children with existing *Ascaris lumbricoides* (an intestinal worm) infection and household access to running water.

Study design

There are several methodological components that need to be considered when planning a study. A study protocol is prepared in advance to define the methods to be used in implementing the study, and in collecting and analysing the data. In this chapter we consider the key components of any study protocol.

Sampling

Epidemiological investigations are undertaken using a **sample population** (of individuals, villages, schools, hospitals, etc.) and findings are then extrapolated to the **target population** (e.g. infants, students, women over 55 years, etc.). In Chapter 4 you learned about the roles of chance and selection bias, and the need for the study sample population to be *representative* of the target general population. We can reduce the role of chance by having a sufficiently large **sample size**. We can reduce selection bias by selecting a random sample from the study population, taking care to ensure that hard-to-reach or minority groups are proportionately sampled.

Sample size

To calculate a sample size, it is necessary to define a specific, testable hypothesis. It is not sufficient to state the association of interest, for example, 'To measure the effect of gender on depression'. Instead we must specify the comparison groups, expected size of the effect, and measure of frequency or association to be detected. This is known as the study objective and would explicitly mention subjects, study population and effect. For example 'To detect a *30% difference* in the *prevalence* of *unipolar depression* between *men* and *women* in *British cities*.'

There are two important concepts in sample size calculation: statistical **power** and **precision**. Statistical power is the probability of detecting an effect if it is real. Statistical precision is the probability of detecting an effect if it is *not* real, i.e. by chance (see Chapter 4 on P-values). It is typical to aim for a sample size with 80–90% power and

5% precision (significance) to detect a valid estimate of effect. Increased power and precision require increasingly larger sample sizes, and this will have implications for how much a study costs and how long it takes.

The size of effect to be detected will also determine the sample size. The larger the effect, the easier it is to detect and the fewer study subjects are required to obtain statistical significance. However, it is rare to find very large effects, so we need to decide what magnitude of effect would be of public health importance. If we found that people drinking one glass of orange juice a day had a 10% reduced risk of catching a cold, we would not recommend that everybody drank orange juice. However, if we found that one glass of orange juice per day reduced the risk of colds by 50%, we might promote it or at least undertake more research into the nature of the relationship.

When calculating a sample size we need to identify the unit of observation: individual, household, school, community, hospital, district, etc. Note, a comparison of improved cognitive function in 500 students taking omega-3 supplementation and 500 students taking a placebo, is not the same as comparing it in 5 exposed schools and 5 unexposed schools each with 100 students. This is because there are likely to be unmeasured similarities between students in the same school that we would not be able to adjust for in the analysis.

Sample size formulae vary according to the outcome of interest (prevalence, incidence, mean) and the level of observation (individual, group). Formulae are available in several statics textbooks (e.g. Kirkwood and Sterne 2003) and computer statistical software packages (e.g. Stata, SPSS) are generally used for sample size calculation.

Sampling methods

Once the sample size has been determined, it is necessary to sample (i.e. select study participants from) the population, with an equal probability of sampling any subject (e.g. individual, household, clinic). Random sampling requires a sampling frame (i.e. a list detailing all eligible subjects in the study population) from which to sample the following:

1   *Simple random sampling* is **random selection** from the sampling frame, for example, by labelling a card for each district, shuffling them and choosing the required number for the study. Random number tables can also reduce selection bias, either by manual or computer-assisted selection depending on sample size.
2   *Systematic sampling* is the selection of sampling units at regular intervals, rather than at random. This may be used when a fixed proportion, e.g. 20%, of the village households, are to be sampled. For example, the starting house may be selected at random, and then a bottle is spun and the fifth house in that direction is also sampled, and the procedure is repeated until sufficient households are recruited.

If a sampling frame is difficult to obtain, if the population is spread out over a large area or if there are subgroups, the following more complex methods may be used:

1   *Stratified sampling* is used when there are distinct groups or strata with different expected frequencies of the outcome or exposure of interest (e.g. age, gender, or other potential confounders). To ensure that the sample represents the population, an equal proportion is sampled from each strata using simple random sampling.
2   *Multi-stage sampling* uses the organizational structure of the study population, with a sampling frame required only for the higher-level unit, and for the primary

sampling units within those higher levels sampled. For example, in a study of school children (i.e. primary sampling units), first *x* number of schools will be randomly sampled from a regional list, and then *y* number of children will be randomly sampled from within each selected school. If the schools are of different sizes, then sampling is carried out using 'probability proportional to size', such that a school with three times as many pupils will be sampled three times more than another school.

3 *Cluster sampling* also uses the organizational structure, but samples all or most of the primary sampling units. An equal probability of sampling the higher-level units is used, regardless of differences in size. For example, in an intervention study of the protective effect of insecticide-treated mosquito nets, where the intervention is known to protect other household members, *x* number of households (i.e. higher-level unit) would be sampled, and all eligible household members (i.e. primary sampling units) within sampled houses would be included in the sample.

Selection criteria

The sample population should represent the general population to whom the results will be applied. However, in some cases it is necessary to exclude certain individuals (e.g. those who may be at greater risk of loss-to-follow-up). It is therefore important to develop clear inclusion and exclusion criteria. **Inclusion criteria** specify the sample population of interest. For example, a study of diabetes in pregnancy may specify 'women enrolled in their first trimester of pregnancy' to obtain sufficient baseline data. Exclusion criteria specify those individuals who are not eligible for inclusion in the study, perhaps because they have underlying conditions that may interfere with assessment of the outcome. For example, in a study of the incidence of clinical malaria fevers, children with severe anaemia (haemoglobin < 5g/dl) at baseline may be excluded because they require medical treatment and may be more prone to a severe outcome.

Informed consent

Ethical permission will need to be obtained from institutional and national ethical bodies before starting any epidemiological studies (and often prior to obtaining funding). For large-scale field trials it is appropriate to inform local government and civil society, and community sensitization meetings may improve local understanding of the study aims and thus cooperation with investigators and recruitment to the study.

Before participants are recruited into an epidemiological study, they must be made fully aware of what the study is about and what the potential risks are. Participants then need to give their consent to participate. This is known as **informed consent**. Sometimes it is not possible for the participant to provide their consent, for example, in the case of a child or an unconscious patient, in which case consent must be obtained from a parent, caregiver or close relative. The information must be provided in the language of the consent giver and, if they are illiterate, the information must be clearly read to them. Consent usually takes the form of a signature, or a fingerprint in the case of illiterate consent givers. Details of the format of information and consent should be clearly stated when the results of the trial are reported.

It is also important that individuals are allowed to refuse to participate and that participants have the option to drop out of the study at any time, without any adverse consequences for their access to preventive or treatment services.

Activity 5.2

1 In a region of country X, all single births occurring in four randomly selected districts during a one-week period were identified from a birth register to assess the gender ratio. What was the outcome measure, what type of sampling was used and what were the inclusion criteria?

2 In a large secondary school with 9 classes of children aged 9–12 years old, 100 girls were randomly selected from the class-registers to be tested for rubella antibodies. What was the outcome measure, what type of sampling was used and what were the inclusion criteria?

3 In country Y, six of 15 regions were randomly selected. Five per cent of households were subsequently selected from each of these six regions and a survey on access to healthcare among children under 5 years of age administered. What was the outcome measure, what type of sampling was used and what were the inclusion criteria?

Data collection

The key to conducting a good epidemiological investigation is to plan the data collection and the analytical approach beforehand. Even studies with large sample sizes and unbiased subject selection can be seriously flawed if key data (e.g. confounders) are not collected. The methods used to collect the data will depend on the exposures and outcomes being studied and how practical and costly it is to collect them. Data may be quantitative (i.e. measurable and relating to 'what?', 'where?' and 'when?') or qualitative (i.e. descriptive and relating to 'why?' and 'how?').

Data may be obtained from sources of routinely collected information on outcomes or exposures (e.g. medical records, census data, health surveys, cancer registries, records kept by schools or employers). These indirect data collection methods have the advantage that the data are already available and can provide information relatively quickly and cheaply. However, data quality may be poor due to missing or inaccurate data. Routine data systems are designed to serve other objectives, such as surveillance, and not a research study, so may not be able to provide all the information required. Therefore, a combination of data collection methods may be used.

Most epidemiological studies obtain data directly from the study participants (or their caregivers). *Direct data collection methods* include questionnaires (e.g. self-administered, filled in by an investigator), structured interviews (e.g. conducted face-to-face, by telephone) and clinical examination (e.g. having a blood sample taken for a diagnostic test). The advantage of direct data collection is that it is collected prospectively (even though questions may relate to historical events) and questionnaires are designed for the specific study. However, in addition to being costly and time-consuming, there may be recall bias or a poor response rate.

Environmental data can also be collected, and the recent advancements in global positioning system (GPS) technology enable us to identify the precise geographic location of a household, village or health centre, for example. Specific data may be collected during an epidemiological study, or from routine sources of climate data (e.g. rainfall, cloud cover), satellite images (e.g. land-use, road access), etc. Whereas John Snow used a simple spot map to identify the cause of the cholera outbreak in 1854 (see Chapter 1), such data can now be analysed using more sophisticated digital technology. Different layers of data (e.g. geographical, epidemiological) can be linked using geographic information systems (GIS), using the location of the data in space and time. This allows a more complex analysis of the data, enabling us to measure the incidence of childhood cancer in relation to distance to the nearest electricity pylon, or the prevalence of malaria infection in relation to altitude and rainfall, for example.

Qualitative methods of direct data collection in epidemiological research may take different forms. Structured interviews can include quantitative or qualitative data. They provide a framework for the interviewer, defining the wording and question sequence to improve the validity of responses. Other qualitative methods such as semi-structured interviews, participant observation or focus group discussions, rarely include quantitative data, and usually deal with limited numbers or non-randomly selected participants, making them inappropriate for the measurement of epidemiological associations. The utility of such methods will depend on the culture and sensitivity of the topic.

Unique identifiers

Investigators must be able to link all necessary data to the appropriate study participant, using a relational database, which is a method of relating different layers of data. A study using multi-stage or cluster sampling will need to collect and link data on the different sampling levels. A cohort study will repeatedly measure individuals, such as the baseline measurement and final contact recording the outcome. In addition to names being common or misspelled, they should not be used, as the identity of participants should be kept confidential and results must always be reported anonymously.

Unique identifiers should be created for each sampling unit (e.g. individual, household, hospital) and used whenever data are collected. For example, a cohort study of malaria in children will include a unique identifier per child (e.g. number 00142) and then collect data on the child (e.g. name, date of birth, gender), the child's household (e.g. household size, distance to nearest health facility), and health facility visits (e.g. data of outpatient attendance, body temperature, haemoglobin level, presence of malaria parasites). Different data collection tools may be used for each layer of data, but all (e.g. household questionnaire, clinic record, blood slide) must record the same unique identifier that will enable, for example, a laboratory test result to be linked to the correct patient.

Data management

It is important that data collection is standardized and investigators ensure the *validity* of the methods used (i.e. that they really are measuring what they aim to measure). Data collection tools need to be carefully designed and pre-tested ('piloted') to reduce data errors. Data format and the legitimate values or ranges for quantitative data need to be defined when developing data collection tools and training those collecting data. Data collection tools include questionnaires, specimen labels for clinical samples and audio/video recordings for qualitative data.

Data may be recorded on paper and entered into a computer, or may be directly entered into a computer or hand-held digital device. When data are being transferred from paper to a computer, it is advisable to double-enter the data to reduce data-entry inputting errors. The computer programme should also be designed to restrict entry only to feasible response values, e.g. prevent the entry of gender as anything other than 'male', 'female' or 'unknown'.

The data should be 'cleaned' periodically. This refers to checking the data to ensure that there are no impossible values (e.g. 50-year-old infants), to check for missing values, and to ensure that data can be linked (e.g. every participant enrolled has an outcome measure).

Data variables

The term 'variable' refers to quantitative data that can have more than one value, and is usually applied to each distinct unit of data that is collected. There are three types of quantitative variable:

1 Binomial variables only have two values (e.g. Yes/No, Male/Female).
2 Categorical variables have several values (e.g. age groups: 0–4 years, 5–9 years, 10–14 years; religion: Christian, Muslim, Jewish, etc.).
3 Continuous variables can have any value within a given range (e.g. blood pressure; age in years, months, or days).

Continuous variables can be grouped into categories, and categorical variables can be further grouped into binary variables. This increases the sample size in each category, providing greater *statistical power* to detect any effect. For example, haemoglobin concentration is a continuous variable, which can be grouped categorically as mild (8–11 g/dl), moderate (5–8 g/dl) or severe (<5 g/dl) anaemia. It can also be grouped binomially as moderately anaemic (<8 g/dl): Yes/No, for example. If qualitative data are used to define outcomes or exposures (e.g. a case-control study of post-natal depression and a history of depression), these will need to be coded as binomial or categorical variables to measure the epidemiological association.

Data analysis

Data may be summarized according to the variable type. Binary and categorical variables may be summarized as proportions of the total (e.g. 49% male and 51% female). Continuous variables are usually presented as the average value of the variable and the amount of variation around this average. This may be summarized as a mean (sum of values divided by the number of values) and standard deviation, or median (midpoint of ordered values) and interquartile range (25–75%, i.e. middle 50% of ordered values). Such summary values are used to present the baseline characteristics of the study sample, to compare exposed with unexposed groups, or to compare cases with controls.

Descriptive data may be presented graphically. In epidemiology, histograms (see Figure 5.1a) are most commonly used to describe the distribution of a continuous outcome, while bar charts (see Figure 5.1b) are used to compare the mean or proportional distribution of a variable by categories. Analytical data may also be presented

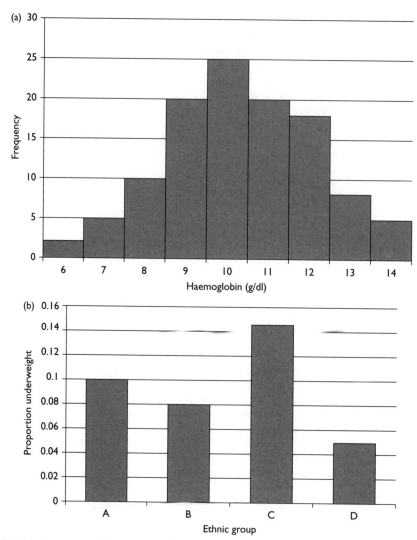

Figure 5.1 (a) Histogram of the frequency distribution of haemoglobin concentration (g/dl) values from a cross-sectional survey of children. (b) Bar chart of the proportion of children in a refugee camp underweight by ethnic group

Source: Ilona Carneiro.

graphically, most commonly as a scatter plot (see Figure 5.2) when investigating the relationship between two continuous variables.

In Chapters 2 and 3 you saw how to present measures of frequency for the outcome of interest and measures of association for the effect of interest. Statistical tests (e.g. chi-squared test or *t*-test) that will not be described here are used to test the **null hypothesis**. This is the opposite of the hypothesis being tested, i.e. that there is *no association* between the exposure and outcome. The *P*-value represents the probability that an association at least as big as the one observed could have occurred by chance alone, if there truly was no association.

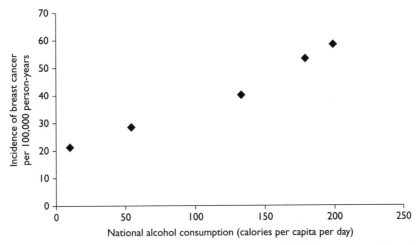

Figure 5.2 Scatter plot of national incidence of breast cancer per 100,000 person-years, by estimated per capita alcohol consumption for selected countries

Source: Drawn by Ilona Carneiro using selected data from Schatzkin et al. (1989).

Regression models

These analyses can also be undertaken using more complex statistical methods known as regression models, which cannot be described in detail here. Briefly, regression is a way of describing the relationship between a variable and potential explanatory factors; in epidemiology this is usually the relationship between an outcome and an exposure or confounding factors. Regression models use data on the explanatory factors to predict the outcome (for further information see Kirkwood and Sterne 2003).

Continuous variables, such as blood pressure or haemoglobin concentration, may be analysed using linear regression, with the results presented as a mean and standard deviation. Binary variables (e.g. prevalence, risk) can be analysed using logistic regression with results presented as an odds ratio. While this is frequently used, it must be remembered that this is only valid for rare outcomes, where the prevalence or risk are approximately equal to the odds (see Chapter 3: Comparability of measures of association on p. 31). Incidence rates may be analysed using other regression models (i.e. Poisson, negative binomial) with results presented as an incidence rate ratio. Categorical variables can be included as explanatory variables in a model but not as outcome variables, so an outcome such as the Glasgow coma score (a neurological scale of consciousness ranging from 3–15) would need to be reclassified as a binary variable and analysed using logistic regression.

If an exposure variable has more than two categories (e.g. ethnicity), we would need to decide which to use as the **reference category** to compare the other categories against. For example, for a quantitative variable such as exposure to smoking, non-smokers may be used as the reference or unexposed group, and other categories (e.g. ex-smokers, infrequent smokers, frequent smokers) can each be treated as the exposed group in turn. For a qualitative variable, such as religion, the choice of reference category is arbitrary. A categorical exposure will result in several relative risks, and you will see the relative risk for the reference category presented as 1.00 (i.e. frequency in unexposed divided by frequency in unexposed). Differences between non-reference categories can be assessed by comparing their 95% confidence intervals: if they overlap, then there is no significant difference at the $P = 0.05$ level. If the exposure can be quantified (e.g. low, medium or high alcohol consumption), the relative risks are examined for a dose–response effect.

Univariate regression analyses the effect of just one explanatory variable and the measures of frequency or association from univariate regression analysis are called 'unadjusted'. The real benefit of regression models is in multivariate regression, which enables us to look at the effect of several variables at the same time and therefore control for other risk factors and confounders. The measures of frequency or association from multivariate regression are 'adjusted' for all the variables included in the model.

If the measure of association varies across categories of a third variable, this is known as **interaction** or **effect modification** because it modifies the effect of the exposure of interest. For example, if the relative risk of ischaemic heart disease in heavy smokers compared to non-smokers is greater at younger ages than at older ages, we would say that age-group was an *effect modifier*, or that there was an *interaction* between age and smoking exposure.

Meta-analysis

When several studies of the same exposure–outcome association are available, it may be possible to obtain a combined estimate effect. A *meta-analysis* uses complex statistical techniques to estimate a combined effect from several studies on the assumption that, despite study differences, the increased statistical power will provide an estimate closer to the true value. A systematic literature review is conducted to identify all published and unpublished records of relevant studies. Predefined inclusion and exclusion criteria are used to select studies of sufficiently good quality and where the methodological differences are not too extreme. In its most simple form, a meta-analysis weights the individual estimates in relation to the sample size of each study. The results of a meta-analysis are usually presented graphically in a forest plot (see Figure 5.3) showing the spread of estimates of effect from individual studies together with the combined estimate of effect. A meta-analysis may be especially useful when faced with conflicting evidence from different studies.

Dissemination of results

As epidemiological studies involve the participation of human subjects, there is a duty to disseminate the results of these studies not only to the scientific and public health communities, but also to those individuals and communities participating in the studies. This may be done through leaflets for participants, community meetings, health education campaigns or providing information to support groups (e.g. Parkinson's Disease Society). It may also be appropriate to present the results to ministries of health or local policy-makers and implementers. The dissemination of study findings should be planned from the beginning, as this helps to focus the study on obtaining information that will be relevant to the end-user.

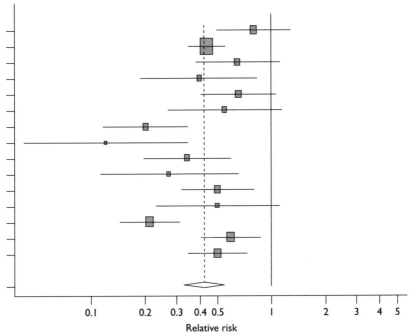

Figure 5.3 Forest plot of estimates from 15 studies of the relative risk of heterosexual HIV infection among circumcised males compared with uncircumcised males. The shaded square and horizontal line correspond to the relative risk and 95% confidence interval for each study. The area of the shaded square reflects the weight of each study. The diamond represents the estimate of combined relative risk and 95% confidence interval

Source: Weiss et al. (2000).

Activity 5.3

For each of the following studies identify the study design, the outcome and exposure of interest, and state whether the variables are binary, categorical, continuous or qualitative. List potential confounders for which you might also want to collect data.

1 The caregivers of 500 children were invited to participate in an epidemiological study by bringing the children for testing for malaria parasites at a central point during a 5-day period. Caregivers were asked about the number of mosquito nets in the household and other information.
2 17,530 men working in the British civil service were surveyed about their grade of employment (e.g. administrative, executive, clerical) and then followed-up for seven and a half years, during which there were 1,086 deaths.
3 Investigators observed and recorded whether the prescribing practice of ten doctors to each of ten patients with respiratory tract infections was consistent with national guidelines on antibiotic prescription. They then assessed whether symptoms had resolved in these 100 patients at a home follow-up visit after 15 days.

4 80 women with breast cancer and their twin sisters without breast cancer were questioned about their previous history and length of oral contraception use.

Conclusion

In this chapter you have reviewed the characteristics of each of the main epidemiological study designs. You have been introduced to the basics of sample selection, sample size calculation, data collection and analysis. These issues will be discussed further in subsequent chapters on specific study designs, and should be considered when critically reviewing any epidemiological data.

References

Doll R and Hill AB (1950) Smoking and carcinoma of the lung; preliminary report. British Medical Journal 2: 739–48.

Kirkwood BR and Sterne JAC (2003) Essential Medical Statistics. Oxford: Blackwell Science.

Schatzkin A, Piantadosi S, Miccozzi M and Bartee D (1989) Alcohol consumption and breast cancer: a cross-national correlation study. International Journal of Epidemiology 18: 28–31.

Schulz KF and Grimes DA (2002) Case-control studies: research in reverse. Lancet 359: 431–4.

Weiss HA, Quigley MA and Hayes RJ (2000) Male circumcision and risk of HIV infection in sub-Saharan Africa: a systematic review and meta-analysis. AIDS 14: 2361–70.

Feedback on activities

Activity 5.1

1 This is case-control study, with twice as many controls as cases. Study participants are identified in relation to their outcome status, although we are not told how controls were selected. The odds ratio of exposure is the only measure of association that can be calculated for a case-control study.

2 This is a cohort study, which would prospectively measure the incidence of heart disease in relation to various exposures recorded at the start of the study. As this is a follow-up study, the incidence will be measured, so that either the risk ratio, odds ratio or incidence rate ratio could be calculated. Given the high likelihood of loss-to-follow-up for a ten-year study, the most appropriate measure would be the incidence rate ratio, if person-time at risk has been sufficiently recorded.

3 This is an intervention study, using untreated mosquito nets as the control for the intervention of treated mosquito nets. We are not told whether it is a randomized trial, or whether observers or participants are blinded to the outcome. The frequency measure is prevalence of anaemia, therefore the appropriate measure of association would be the prevalence ratio.

4 This is an ecological study, comparing the incidence of infant mortality with exposure to gross domestic product, an indicator of standard of living at a population (national) level. The measure of frequency is incidence, however, there is no measure of person-time at risk. The preferred measure of association would be the risk ratio, although the odds ratio could also be calculated.

5 This is a cross-sectional study measuring existing (prevalent) infections, and therefore prevalence ratio will be the appropriate measure of association between household access to running water and ascaris infection.

Activity 5.2

1 The outcome measure of interest would be prevalence of males (or females). This is
a cluster sample, with all births in a defined period being sampled for each selected
district. The inclusion criteria would be all single births, i.e. multiple births (twins,
triplets, etc.) would be excluded.

2 The outcome measure of interest would be the prevalence of rubella seropositivity
(proportion with rubella antibodies). Simple random sampling was used, as the girls
could have been from any of the nine eligible classes. The inclusion criteria would be
girls, aged 9–12 years old, providing informed (parental) consent (as blood samples
would need to be taken).

3 The outcome measure of interest would be access to healthcare (e.g. percentage
of children taken to a health clinic with 48 hours of fever onset). This is a multi-stage
sample. First, the regions were selected by simple random sampling, and then
5% of households in each region were selected, such that larger regions would
contribute more households to the study sample. Inclusion criteria would be
households with at least one child under 5 years old and consenting to participate in
the survey.

Activity 5.3

1 This is a cross-sectional study of the relationship between malaria prevalence and
household mosquito net ownership. Prevalence is a binary outcome, while number
of mosquito nets is a continuous exposure (depending on household size), which
could be regrouped as categorical (e.g. 0, 1–2, 3+) or binary (i.e. 0, 1+). The measure
of association would be the prevalence ratio.

  Potential confounders should include socio-economic indicators that are likely to
affect mosquito net ownership and prevalence of malaria.

2 This is an occupational cohort study measuring the relationship between employment grade and incidence of all-cause death. The exposure is categorical, and the
outcome could be binary (risk of death) or continuous (mortality rate, if the person-
time at risk is known for each individual). The measure of association would be a risk
ratio or incidence rate ratio.

  Likely measurable confounders are smoking history, medical conditions, blood
pressure, body-mass-index (weight divided by height-squared), etc.

3 This is a cohort study following-up participants to measure the 'risk' of cure, which
is a binary outcome. The explanatory variable is qualitative and was measured using
participant observation. It would need to be coded as binary (e.g. according to guidelines, not according to guidelines) or categorical (e.g. number of guideline points
met). Presumably many more than ten patient consultations would be observed in
order to avoid observer influence and to recruit ten patients with respiratory tract
infections). The measure of association would be a risk ratio.

  Confounders would relate to differences between the prescribing doctors and
their practices that might also affect patients' risk of cure. For example, a more
onscientious doctor who might prescribe correctly, might also be more likely to
explain medication instructions, antibiotic compliance and second-line measures

to the patient. Likewise, a busy doctor in an under-resourced neighbourhood may make more prescribing mistakes and the patients may have poorer general health.

4 This is a *matched* case-control study, where each breast cancer case is individually matched with a control on the basis of genetics, age and some socio-behavioural factors. The outcome is binomial (cancer or no cancer), and the explanatory variable may be continuous (number of years of contraceptive use) or categorical (e.g. none, <2 years, 2–5 years, 5–10 years, 10+ years of contraceptive use). The measure of association will be the odds ratio of *exposure*, as this is a case-control study.

Age, family history of breast cancer, and ethnicity have already been controlled for. Potential confounders that may be associated with length of contraceptive use and risk of breast cancer include parity (i.e. number of live births), breast-feeding practices, onset of menopause, alcohol use and physical activity.

Ecological studies 6

Overview

Ecological studies *analyse* epidemiological associations at a *population* or group level, usually using data collected for other purposes. While the ecological design is relatively convenient and inexpensive, it is subject to many biases. In this chapter you will review the characteristics, advantages and limitations of the ecological study design for analytical epidemiology. You will be introduced to different sources of routine data, and methods of standardization to compare data from populations with different demographic structures.

Learning objectives

When you have completed this chapter you should be able to:

* describe the features and uses of ecological studies
* identify different sources of routine data that may be used
* define and calculate standardized rates, using direct or indirect methods, to compare populations
* discuss the potential sources of bias and confounding in ecological studies.

What defines an ecological study?

Ecological studies *analyse the relationship between outcome and exposure at a population level*, where 'population' represents a group of individuals with a shared characteristic such as geography, ethnicity, socio-economic status or employment. The defining factor of an ecological study is that data on both outcome and exposure are not linked to, and usually not available for, *individual* study participants. The unit of analysis is the group, and outcome and exposure are summarized at the group level. For example, the incidence rates of an outcome in two groups are compared with the proportion of each group exposed to a potential risk factor.

Advantages and disadvantages

The main reasons for undertaking an ecological study are as follows:

1 When data are only available at a group level, or differences may vary more between groups/areas than within groups/areas (e.g. air pollution, healthcare services, and climate variation between regions).

2 If data are difficult to measure at an individual level, for example, because of considerable variation in individual dietary habits, group averages may be easier to distinguish (e.g. ethnic or social differences in alcohol consumption may be more
consistent than individual measures).

3 To study group-specific effects where interventions may be aimed at the group level
through control programmes, health policies or legislation, such as injury prevention
through national road safety laws.

4 When data are readily available (faster and less expensive to collect) at a group level,
as with indirect data sources from routine monitoring, population registries, demographic surveys or censuses.

However, because the data on exposure and outcome are not linked at the individual
level, it is not possible to infer causality. This design suffers from many potential biases
(see Interpretation section on p. 85). It may also be necessary to standardize data (see
Analysis section on p. 80) if the groups being compared have different demographic
characteristics (e.g. age distribution).

Study design

An ecological study may compare populations or groups using a *multi-group design*,
periods of time using a *time-trend design*, or groups and time using a *mixed design*. In a
multi-group study, data on the frequency of an outcome may be measured individually
and aggregated (combined), or estimated for particular groups (e.g. country, district,
hospital). Similarly, individual-level data on exposures are aggregated for the same
groups. The relationship between outcome and various exposures are then compared
at this group level to see if an association can be found. Figure 6.1 shows that the

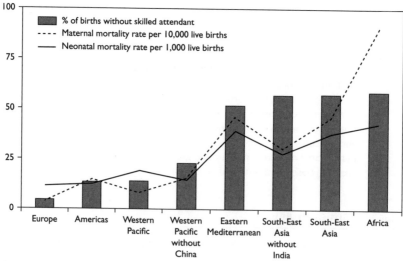

Figure 6.1 Incidence of neonatal and maternal mortality by percentage of births without a skilled birth
attendant for different regions

Source: WHO (2005).

incidence of neonatal and maternal mortality for each WHO region increases with the percentage of births without a skilled birth attendant. This design is often used to compare spatial (geographical) patterns in the frequency of an outcome. For example, by comparing the geographical distribution of populations with high frequency genetic blood disorders (e.g. thalassaemia) with that of malaria, it was suggested that such genes might provide some protection against malaria infection. The use of geographical information systems (see Chapter 5) has enabled more sophisticated analyses of environmental risks for health outcomes.

In a time-trend study, data on outcome and exposure for a given population are compared over a period of time. Comparisons can investigate whether changes in incidence of an outcome over time correlate with changes in risk factors or coverage of an intervention over the same period (e.g. changes in air quality and incidence of asthma in children). However, if the outcome has a long or unknown **latent** period (i.e. where it is present but not yet detected), time-trend analysis may be difficult to interpret. In addition, it is possible that the association between exposure and outcome may vary over time, making interpretation of a time-trend analysis more complicated.

Mixed-studies compare different groups over time, and if consistent differences are seen this may lend weight to a causal association, as in Bradford-Hill's considerations for causality (see Chapter 4).

Sampling

The choice of study sample in ecological studies is often defined by availability and quality of routinely collected data. For example, hospital records may vary according to institution, and using these to compare outcome frequencies for different hospital catchment areas will subject the analysis to inherent selection and information bias of each hospital's record-keeping systems.

Data collection

Data may be measured:

1 at an individual level and aggregated at a group level, such as data on cancer incidence from a cancer registry, or all-cause mortality rates from consecutive censuses.
2 at a group level but vary by individual, such as estimated neonatal and maternal mortality rates, and percentage of births without a skilled birth attendant by WHO region (see Figure 6.1).
3 at a group level as they are attributes of the group and do not vary by individual, such as national estimates of life expectancy and gross domestic product (see Figure 6.2).

Routine data sources

Many ecological studies utilize data collected routinely for other purposes, as these are readily available at little or no cost. Routine data often provide baseline information to describe a population, and variations in health outcome (e.g. by age, sex, ethnicity, geography). If routine data are collected systematically over time, we can study the

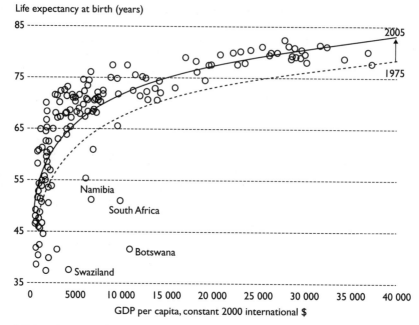

Figure 6.2 Gross Domestic Product (GDP) per capita and life expectancy at birth in 169 countries (1975 and 2005)

Source: WHO (2008).

progression of an outcome in a population or the impact of a health intervention such as screening or vaccination.

However, the accuracy of such data depends on the infrastructure available to collect them and how they are used. The more often a data source is used, the greater the incentive to ensure that data are complete, valid and accurate. Routine data sources include:

1 demographic data through population censuses and household surveys;
2 births and deaths through vital registration systems or demographic surveillance systems;
3 information on chronic conditions through outcome-specific registries.

Demographic data

Demographic data describe the basic characteristics of a population, such as age, gender, ethnic group, religion and socio-economic indicators. Many countries collect demographic data through regular population censuses. A census is the systematic collection of data about all members of a population, as opposed to a sample, at one time-point using a cross-sectional design. While in high-income countries censuses may take the form of postal questionnaires, countries without sufficient infrastructure require census staff to undertake door-to-door visits. A full population census is ideally carried out at regular intervals (e.g. every ten years), however, given its complexity and cost, this is not always possible. Census data may also be used to provide data on fertility, mortality and key health indices in countries with poor *vital registration* (see below).

Censuses provide data on the demographic structure of a population that are needed for data standardization (see Analysis section on p. 80). The World Health Organization (WHO) publishes estimates of population size and key health indicators for its 193 member states on the Internet (World Health Organization 2011). While these may not be as detailed as some locally collected data, it does enable us to make national comparisons.

Population health surveys are also conducted by some countries to provide information on specific demographic groups or health outcomes. UNICEF undertakes Multiple Indicator Cluster Surveys to provide information on health indicators. Demographic and Health Surveys (DHS) collect nationally representative data from household surveys in developing countries using standardized methodologies and data collection methods. These data are also publicly available (Measure DHS 2011) and can be used to form the basis for ecological studies comparing national or sub-national populations, or to show changes in health outcomes over time in response to changing exposures and public health interventions.

Vital registration data

Many countries collect data on births and deaths by age, sex and cause through an official birth and death certification, known as civil registration. Birth data may be used as a health outcome or to provide a denominator for mortality. Death data may be used as an outcome, or as an indicator of population health and the provision of medical care to large populations, i.e. as an exposure. The main indicators used for national and sub-national analyses are neonatal (first 28 days of life), infant (1–11 months of age) and under-five (<5 years of age) and maternal mortality per 1,000 (or 100,000) live births. Note that while these are often called rates, they are actually risks (see Chapter 2). For example, infant mortality in Mozambique fell from 155 per 1,000 live births in 1990 to 96 per 1,000 in 2009. This decline may be interpreted as evidence of improvements in medical care, sanitation and housing in Mozambique between 1990 and 2009.

Cause-specific mortality statistics are usually based on identifying a single underlying (primary) cause of death, defined as the 'disease or injury that initiated the series of events leading directly to death, or the circumstances of the accident or violence that produced the fatal injury'. In addition to the underlying cause of death, data is also recorded on significant conditions or diseases, for example, diabetes, which may have contributed to death.

These data allow comparison of mortality within countries, over time, and with other countries if the same definitions are used. To enable comparisons to be made, a single standardized coding system is used when death certificates are collated. Trained personnel use the International Classification of Disease (ICD), the tenth version of which came into use in 1994, to code cause of death. However, there may be *information bias* related to the accuracy of clinical diagnoses, completion of the registration of death, or the subsequent coding. For example, outcomes that are stigmatized (e.g. maternal death due to illegal abortion, suicide, HIV/AIDS) may not be accurately reported. All these factors need to be considered when using and interpreting these data.

The WHO collates data on registered deaths by age group, sex, year and cause of death for individual member states as part of its mandate to provide health information worldwide (World Health Organization 2011). However, the proportion of deaths that are registered in a population will be lower in settings with weaker infrastructure for certification and collation of data on numbers and causes of death. The 'completeness' of mortality data will depend on access to formal health services, and is likely to be less in low-income countries and rural areas. Some countries use sample vital registration to collate data on births, all-cause deaths and cause-specific deaths in a nationally representative sample of population clusters, to obtain data that can then be extrapolated to national level. In some countries, demographic surveillance sites collect vital registration data on a defined population. While these may not be nationally representative, they may provide useful indications of trends over time, and may be used for ecological analyses of risk factors.

Disease registries

Data from disease registries are frequently used in ecological studies for comparison of trends over time, and comparison between populations within a country and between countries with similar registration systems. These will be discussed in more detail in Chapter 12, as they are also used for surveillance.

Analysis

In ecological studies, measures of exposure and outcome are often continuous (e.g. disease prevalence, mortality rate, proportion of population exposed to a particular factor, mean temperature in a geographical region). Such data need to be displayed as a scatter plot (see Figure 6.2) in which the outcome variable is plotted against the exposure variable. From this we can determine whether there seem to be any trends in the data, which can then be confirmed using statistical methods (correlation or regression models). Correlation measures how closely two variables are associated, while regression describes the relationship mathematically, enabling the prediction of one variable from another (for further information, see Kirkwood and Sterne 2003). Alternatively, if the outcome can be grouped as two comparison groups, we can estimate the relative risk of outcome for a given exposure. Regression models can then be used to estimate the relative risk for continuous exposures and adjust for potential confounders.

Standardization

In an ecological study, the data may come from different places (e.g. countries, regions within a country) or from the same population during different time-periods. Comparing the *crude* incidence rate of an outcome may result in significant confounding if there are differences in the age-structure or other demographic characteristics (e.g. gender, ethnic group) between these different data sources. For example, Figure 6.3 shows that the male population of South Africa has many more children and young people than elderly, whilst Switzerland has a more middle-aged and older population. Age standardization will be described here to overcome such differences, although the same methods can be applied to standardization for other demographic characteristics.

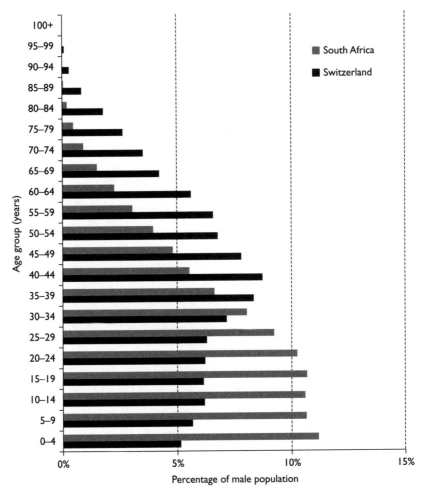

Figure 6.3 Population age-distribution of males in Switzerland and South Africa in 2005
Source: Drawn by Ilona Carneiro using data from United Nations Population Division (2008).

To reduce confounding, we standardize the data by comparing them to a population for which the demographic structure is known ('standard population') using direct or indirect methods. There are available 'standards' based on averages from world or European populations, however, the actual population structure used as the *standard* does not matter, so long as the same structure is used for all populations being compared. This is because the standardized rate that results cannot be used as a real value (i.e. it does not relate to a population, time and place), but only allows us to compare populations and to calculate incidence rate ratios adjusting for differences in their underlying structures.

Direct standardization is used when we know the group-specific outcome rates in the study population. The age-specific rate is the incidence rate (number of cases divided by the person-time at risk) calculated separately for each age group. The percentage of the standard population in each age group is multiplied by the age-specific rate for that age group in the study population to obtain a weighted average. The sum of these across all age groups divided by 100 gives a **standardized rate** for the whole population. The directly standardized rate is therefore the expected rate in the *standard* population if the age-specific rates of the study population had applied.

We will illustrate this with an example. The mortality rate for all cancers in men in 2007 was 246 per 100,000 in Switzerland and 58 per 100,000 in South Africa (World Health Organization 2010). We might calculate the incidence rate ratio as 246 ÷ 58 = 4.24 and conclude that men living in Switzerland have a four times greater risk of dying from cancer than those living in South Africa. Since we know from Figure 6.3 that the age-distribution of these two populations is different, we might want to look more closely at the age-specific rates to see at which ages this huge difference occurs. However, Figure 6.4 suggests that the age-specific rates are actually very similar until old age, at which point men aged over 85 years old have almost twice as much risk of dying of cancer in South Africa than in Switzerland. How can we make sense of these contradictory results?

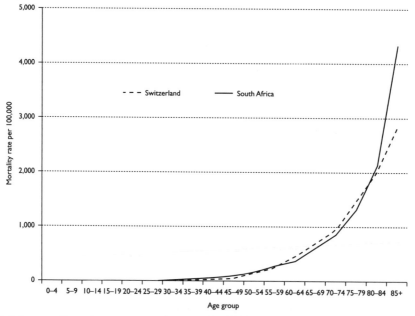

Figure 6.4 Age-specific male cancer mortality rates for 2007 in Switzerland and South Africa
Source: Drawn by Ilona Carneiro using data from WHO cancer mortality database (2010).

To compare these data properly we must standardize the *crude* rates to see how many cancer deaths we might expect if the two populations had the same age-structures. Table 6.1 shows the World Standard Population developed by the WHO and based on the predicted average age structure of the world's population from 2000 to 2025 (Ahmad et al. 2001). Using this, we can calculate the expected cancer mortality rate in each population of interest if they had the same population age-structure.

First, multiply the *study* population age-specific mortality rate by the percentage of the *standard* population for each age group, then sum all of these and divide by 100. The

Table 6.1 Direct standardization of Swiss and South African (SA) 2007 male cancer mortality rates per 100,000

Age group (years)	World standard population (%)	Swiss 2007 age-specific mortality rate*	Expected rate* in Switzerland	SA 2007 age-specific mortality rate*	Expected rate* in SA
0–4	8.86	1.60	14.18	2.70	23.92
5–9	8.69	3.00	26.07	1.80	15.64
10–14	8.60	1.80	15.48	1.80	15.48
15–19	8.47	2.60	22.02	3.40	28.80
20–24	8.22	6.10	50.14	5.50	45.21
25–29	7.93	8.60	68.20	9.10	72.16
30–34	7.61	9.20	70.01	20.10	152.96
35–39	7.15	11.70	83.66	32.70	233.81
40–44	6.59	28.40	187.16	53.50	352.57
45–49	6.04	58.60	353.94	102.70	620.31
50–54	5.37	147.10	789.93	167.70	900.55
55–59	4.55	255.70	1,163.44	279.00	1,269.45
60–64	3.72	452.50	1,683.30	370.10	1,376.77
65–69	2.96	671.40	1,987.34	596.60	1,765.94
70–74	2.21	969.80	2,143.26	860.50	1,901.71
75–79	1.52	1,464.00	2,225.28	1,321.30	2,008.38
80–84	0.91	2,015.30	1,833.92	2,115.30	1,924.92
85+	0.63	2,838.30	1,788.13	4,330.70	2,728.34
Total	100.00		14,505.45		15,436.91

Note: * per 100,000 population

Source: Ilona Carneiro, using data from Ahmad et al. (2001) and WHO cancer mortality database (World Health Organization 2010).

male cancer mortality rate for Switzerland *standardized for age* is 145 per 100,000 and for South Africa is 154 per 100,000. These are similar, indicating that after adjusting for differences in age-structure there is no difference in the overall incidence rate of cancer mortality between these two countries, although the age-specific rates will differ.

Indirect standardization calculates the expected number of cases in the *study* population if the age-specific rates of a 'standard' population had applied. It can be used if we do not have age-specific rates for the study population of interest, but we know the population structure and the total number of cases. The expected number of cases is then used to calculate a **standardized mortality (or morbidity) ratio** (SMR), which compares the observed number of deaths (or poor health outcome) to that expected in the same population. The SMR is interpreted in the same way as a relative risk and is calculated as:

$$\text{Standardized Mortality/Morbidity Ratio} = \frac{\textbf{Observed cases in population of interest}}{\textbf{Expected cases in population of interest}}$$

Using the example above, suppose that we did not have the age-specific mortality rates for Switzerland, but we had this for South Africa. Assuming that the male population age-structure for Switzerland in 2005 (from Figure 6.3) was still valid in 2007, and we knew that there were 8,596 deaths from cancer among men in Switzerland in 2007. We could calculate the expected deaths for each age group by multiplying the population in each age group in Switzerland with the age-specific incidence rate for South Africa (see Table 6.2).

Table 6.2 Indirect age standardization of Swiss and South African (SA) 2007 male cancer mortality

Age group (years)	SA 2007 mortality rate (per 100,000)	Switzerland 2005 population (1,000s)	Expected deaths in Switzerland 2007
0–4	2.70	187	5
5–9	1.80	205	4
10–14	1.80	225	4
15–19	3.40	223	8
20–24	5.50	226	12
25–29	9.10	228	21
30–34	20.10	261	52
35–39	32.70	303	99
40–44	53.50	317	170
45–49	102.70	283	291
50–54	167.70	247	414
55–59	279.00	239	667
60–64	370.10	204	755
65–69	596.60	154	919
70–74	860.50	128	1,101
75–79	1,321.30	97	1,282
80–84	2,115.30	66	1,396
85+	4,330.70	46	1,992
Total		3,639	9,191

Source: Ilona Carneiro, using data from Ahmad et al. (2001) and WHO cancer mortality database (World Health Organization 2010).

If Switzerland had the same age-specific mortality rates as South Africa 2007, we would expect 9,191 cancer deaths among men in 2007. The SMR can then be calculated as 8,596 ÷ 9,191 = 0.94, i.e. nearly one, indicating little difference in male cancer mortality between Switzerland and South Africa in 2007.

SMRs should only be compared with the *standard* population, unless the underlying population structures are shown to be comparable. As the indirect standardization method does not use a common standard age-structure, if SMRs are calculated for several populations with very different age-structures, they must not be compared with each other. This is because any differences may be due to the population structures rather than differences in age-specific rates (i.e. confounding by age).

Interpretation

The results of ecological studies need to be interpreted with caution for the following reasons:

1 **Ecological fallacy:** This is the mismatch that arises from trying to draw conclusions about individual-level epidemiological associations from a group-level study. For example, an ecological analysis of anaemia prevalence and malaria prevalence in children for several districts of country X may reveal that the two are closely related. However, we cannot determine from these data that this relationship exists at an individual level and that children with malaria are the same as those that have anaemia; they may be completely different. Note that the same mismatch can occur when trying to draw conclusions about group-level effects from individual-level data. Therefore, it is not possible to make any causal inference from an ecological study.

2 Bias: Data may be collected in different ways for different groups, and diagnostic criteria and technologies can change over time, leading to differential misclassification (see Chapter 4).

3 Mixing: Geographical comparisons may suffer from migration of populations between groups over the period of the study, which may dilute differences between groups.

4 Confounding: Data are often collected for purposes other than epidemiological research and at a group level data on potential confounding factors are often missing.

Activity 6.1

Table 6.3 shows HIV-related deaths and mid-year population by age group. The mid-year population of country Y in 2010 was estimated at 198,812,000.

Table 6.3 HIV-related deaths and estimated population by age group in country Y, 2010

Age group (years)	HIV-related deaths	Mid-year population
0–4	110	11,217,000
5–14	30	28,146,000
15–24	423	31,698,000
25–34	4,328	37,315,000
35–44	4,096	29,305,000
45–54	1,522	19,276,000
55+	897	41,855,000
Total	11,406	198,812,000

Source: Adapted from Bailey et al. (2005).

1 Calculate the crude HIV-related mortality rate and the age-specific HIV-related mortality rate for country Y in 2010.
2 Compare the HIV-related mortality rate for country Y with an estimated rate of 4 per 100,000 for country Z in 2010 using an appropriate crude (unstandardized) measure of association and interpret your result.
3 Table 6.4 shows the age-specific HIV-related mortality rate for country Z in 2010. Comparing this with the age-specific HIV-related mortality that you calculated for country Y, what do you observe and what might explain this?

Table 6.4 Age-specific HIV-related mortality for country Z in 2010

Age group (years)	Age-specific HIV-related mortality per 100,000
0–4	1.00
5–14	0.14
15–24	1.30
25–34	11.60
35–44	14.00
45–54	7.90
55+	2.10

Source: Adapted from Bailey et al. (2005).

4 The mid-year population for country Z in 2010 was estimated as 240,000,000. Using the information provided, name and calculate a standardized HIV-related mortality measure to compare these two populations, and interpret your result.

Activity 6.2

Table 6.5 compares age-specific mortality in two populations.

Table 6.5 Age-specific mortality rates in City A and City B

Age	City A			City B		
	Deaths	Population (1,000s)	Mortality rate (per 1,000)	Deaths	Population (1,000s)	Mortality rate (per 1,000)
0–17	2,343	2,101	1.10	2,076	440	4.70
18–44	6,104	2,365	2.60	766	256	3.00
45–60	23,845	857	27.80	3,210	96	33.40
60+	38,102	656	58.10	2,311	38	60.80
All	70,394	5,979	11.80	8,363	830	10.10

Source: Bailey et al. (2005).

1 Describe the data in Table 6.5. Can you determine whether mortality rates are higher in City A or City B?

2 Use indirect standardization to calculate the number of deaths you would have expected to see in City B if it had the same age-specific mortality rates as City A.

3 Calculate and interpret the standardized mortality ratio (SMR) for City A compared with City B.

Activity 6.3

An ecological study was conducted to investigate the effect of air pollutants on pregnancy outcomes estimated from routinely collected data (Bobak and Leon 1999). Figure 6.5 shows data on the annual prevalence of low birthweight (<2500g) and

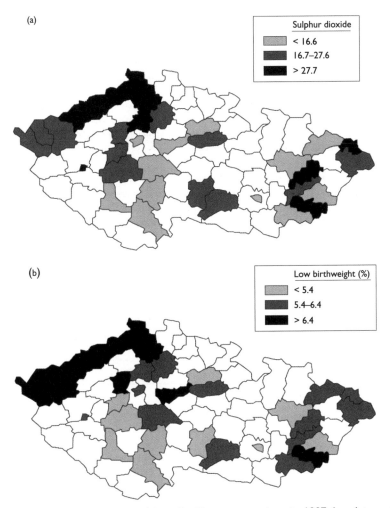

Figure 6.5 (a) Annual geometric mean sulphur dioxide concentrations in 1987 (no data available for unshaded areas). (b) Prevalence of low birthweight (<2500g) in districts for which data were available in (a)
Source: Bobak and Leon (1999).

geometric mean concentration of sulphur dioxide plotted for the 85 administrative districts of the Czech Republic.

1 Looking at Figure 6.5, was there an association between sulphur dioxide concentration and prevalence of low birthweight for the 39 shaded districts?

A logistic regression model was used to estimate associations, adjusting for socio-economic factors at the district level. An odds ratio for low birthweight of 1.10 (95% CI: 1.02, 1.17) and an odds ratio for stillbirths of 0.98 (95% CI: 0.80, 1.20) was estimated for each 50 $\mu g/m^2$ increase in sulphur dioxide pollution.

2 Interpret these results in relation to whether there is an epidemiological association between the exposure and each outcome.

Activity 6.4

Data from a 1976 aerial survey were used to determine the measure of outdoor gamma radiation at the mid-point of each of 69 census areas within a ten-mile radius of a nuclear power station in the USA (Hatch and Susser 1990). Incident cases of cancer between 1 January 1975 and 31 December 1985 were identified from hospital records within a 30-mile radius of the nuclear power station and referral hospitals in nearby cities. The population at risk for each census area was estimated from census data. The incidence rate of cancer in children aged 0–14 years was calculated for each of the 69 census areas.

1 Identify the study hypothesis, exposure and outcome of interest.

The census areas were divided into quartiles (four groups with equal numbers, each representing a quarter of the total sample) based on the level of outdoor gamma radiation. Table 6.6 shows the incidence rate of childhood leukaemia and childhood cancer for each quartile.

Table 6.6 Outdoor gamma radiation and cancer incidence among children from 69 census areas within 10 miles of a US nuclear plant

Incidence per 100,000	Gamma radiation at mid-point of census area			
	Quartile 1	Quartile 2	Quartile 3	Quartile 4
Childhood leukaemia	1.9	1.5	2.0	4.9
Childhood cancer	8.2	15.4	13.9	22.6

Source: Hatch and Susser (1990).

2 Identify and calculate an appropriate measure of relative risk for both childhood leukaemia and all childhood cancers, comparing incidence in those with the highest exposure to gamma radiation (Quartile 4) with incidence in those with the lowest exposure (Quartile 1). Interpret your result.

3 From your calculation and the data presented, can you say that higher exposure to outdoor gamma radiation causes an increased risk of childhood cancers? Give reasons for your answer.

Conclusion

In this chapter you have reviewed key features, advantages and limitations of the eco-logical study design. There are various sources of routinely collected data that may be used in ecological studies, such as vital registrations, population censuses and outcome registries. While this design is generally cost-effective, and is necessary for some population-level risk factors, it is not possible to infer causality at an individual level from the results of ecological studies.

References

Ahmad OB, Boschi-Pinto C, Lopez AD, et al. (2001) Age standardization of rates: a new WHO standard. *GPE Discussion Paper Series*. Geneva: World Health Organization.

Bailey L, Vardulaki K, Langham J and Chandramohan D (2005) *Introduction to Epidemiology*. 1st edn. Maidenhead: Open University Press.

Bobak M and Leon DA (1999) Pregnancy outcomes and outdoor air pollution: an ecological study in districts of the Czech Republic 1986–8. *Occupational and Environmental Medicine* 56: 539–43.

Measure DHS (2011) *Demographic and Health Surveys* [Online]. Available: http://www.measuredhs.com/start.cfm (accessed 02/05/2011).

Hatch M and Susser M (1990) Background gamma radiation and childhood cancers within ten miles of a US nuclear plant. *International Journal of Epidemiology* 19: 546–52.

Kirkwood BR and Sterne JAC (2003) *Essential Medical Statistics*. Oxford: Blackwell Science.

United Nations *World Population Prospects, the 2008 revision* [Online]. Available: http://www.un.org/esa/population/unpop.htm (accessed 01/05/2011).

World Health Organization (2005) *World Health Report 2005: Make Every Mother and Child Count*. Geneva: World Health Organization.

World Health Organization (2008) *The World Health Report 2008: Primary Health Care – Now More Than Ever*. Geneva: World Health Organization.

World Health Organization (2010) *Cancer Mortality Database* [Online]. Available: http://www-dep.iarc.fr/WHOdb/WHOdb.htm (accessed 01/05/2011).

World Health Organization (2011) *Global Health Observatory (GHO)* [Online]. Available: http://www.who./gho/en/ (accessed 02/05/2001).

Feedback for activities

Activity 6.1

1 Mortality rate is simply the incidence rate for deaths, and is calculated as the number of deaths divided by the mid-year population for the time at risk (i.e. the year 2010). For example, for the whole population the number of HIV-related deaths was 11,406 and the mid-year population was 198,812,000. Therefore the crude HIV-related mortality rate was 11,406 ÷ 198,812,000 = 0.000057 or 5.74 per 100,000. The results for age-specific mortality rates are shown in the last column of Table 6.7.

2 The appropriate crude measure of association is the incidence rate ratio (IRR) calculated as the incidence in the exposed divided by the incidence in the unexposed (see Chapter 3).

For HIV-related mortality the IRR for country Y compared with country Z is 5.74 ÷ 4 = 1.44. This might suggest that the all-cause mortality rate in country Y is

Table 6.7 HIV-related deaths and estimated population by age group in country Y, 2010

Age group (years)	HIV-related deaths	Mid-year population	Age-specific HIV-related mortality rate per 100,000
0–4	110	11,217,000	0.98
5–14	30	28,146,000	0.11
15–24	423	31,698,000	1.33
25–34	4,328	37,315,000	11.60
35–44	4,096	29,305,000	13.98
45–54	1,522	19,276,000	7.90
55+	897	41,855,000	2.14
Total	11,406	198,812,000	5.74

Source: Adapted from Bailey et al. (2005).

approximately 44% higher than that in country Z. However, there is no information on how these measures were obtained and therefore we cannot account for the role of chance (no 95% Confidence Intervals are given), bias or confounding.

3 The age-specific HIV-related mortality rates appear to be almost identical in both populations. Given that the crude population rates were different, this would suggest that the population age-structures are different, probably mostly in those age groups at highest risk of HIV.

4 As the age-specific rates are similar, it means that if direct standardization methods were used, the age-standardized rate of HIV-specific mortality would be similar in the two countries. If indirect methods were used, the SMR would equal 1. (You can check this by using the World standard population structure in Table 6.1 or by applying the age-specific rates of country Z to the age-specific population for country Y.)

Activity 6.2

1 Age-specific mortality increases with age in both populations. The crude (whole population) mortality rate is slightly higher in City A than in City B. However, if we look at the age-specific mortality rates, we see that they are higher in all age groups in City B compared with City A.

The higher crude mortality is likely to be due to the population age-structure being older in City A than in City B (10.97% versus 4.58% aged 60+) as the elderly are generally at greater risk of dying. Therefore age acts as a confounder since it is independently associated both with the exposure (living in City A or B) and the outcome (mortality).

2 You should have constructed a table to calculate the number of expected deaths in city B if it had the same age-specific mortality rates as the 'standard' population of City A. Your table should look like Table 6.8 and the total number of expected deaths in City B would be 6,027.

3 Using the expected deaths from Table 6.8, you can calculate the SMR as:

$$\text{SMR} = \frac{\text{Observed deaths}}{\text{Expected deaths}} = \frac{8,363}{6,027} = 1.39$$

Table 6.8 Expected mortality for City B using rates from City A

| | City A | | City B |
Age	Mortality rate (per 1,000)	Population (1,000s)	Deaths expected
0–17	1.10	440	(440,000 × 1.1)/1,000 = 484
18–44	2.60	256	(256,000 × 2.6)/1,000 = 666
45–60	27.80	96	(96,000 × 27.8)/1,000 = 2,669
60	58.10	38	(38,000 × 58.1)/1,000 = 2,208
All	11.80	830	6,027

Source: Natasha Howard.

An SMR of 1.39 tells us that people living in City B are 1.39 times (or 39%) more likely to die than people living in City A.

Activity 6.3

1 The presentation of a map for each variable is descriptive rather than analytical, but we can see that both sulphur dioxide pollution and the prevalence of low birthweight were higher in the north-western and south-eastern districts, although the overlap is not perfect. This suggests that a relationship might exist, but requires an epidemiological analysis of the data.

2 The odds ratio for low birthweight is 1.10, indicating a 10% increase in the annual prevalence of low birthweight for every 50 $\mu g/m^2$ increase in population exposure to sulphur dioxide pollution. The 95% confidence interval was 1.02–1.17, meaning we can be 95% certain that the true estimate of the odds ratio lies within this range. The 95% confidence interval does not include 1.00, meaning that the *P*-value will be less than 5 (i.e. less than 5% chance that this association is not true). However, this does not mean that individual exposure to sulphur dioxide will increase the risk of low birthweight in a pregnant mother.

The odds ratio for stillbirths is 0.98, and the 95% confidence interval includes 1.00, meaning there is no evidence that population exposure to sulphur dioxide pollution affects the risk of stillbirths.

Activity 6.4

1 This is an ecological study as exposure (outdoor gamma radiation) and outcome (incidence rate of childhood cancer) are measured and calculated at the level of the census area. The hypothesis being tested was, therefore, that *populations* (not individuals) exposed to higher levels of outdoor gamma radiation in 1976 would have a higher incidence of childhood cancer between 1975–1985.

2 The appropriate measure of relative risk is the *incidence rate ratio* (see Chapter 3).

Using Quartile 4 as the exposed group and Quartile 1 as the unexposed group, we calculate the incidence rate ratio (IRR) for childhood leukaemia as:

$$\text{IRR for childhood leukaemia} = \frac{4.9}{1.9} = 2.58$$

and the incidence rate ratio for childhood cancer as:

$$\text{IRR for childhood cancer} = \frac{22.6}{8.2} = 2.76$$

An incidence rate ratio of 2.58 for childhood leukaemia and an incidence rate ratio of 2.76 for all childhood cancers indicates these are *more than twice as high* among *populations* exposed to the highest quartile of outdoor gamma radiation, as among populations exposed to the lowest quartile of outdoor gamma radiation, between 1975–1985 in this study population.

3 We can say that the study results show that populations exposed to higher levels of outdoor gamma radiation have higher incidences of childhood cancer.

However, we *cannot* conclude that outdoor gamma radiation is a causal factor for the increased risk of childhood cancer for several reasons:

(a) This is an ecological study, and we do not know that the incident cancer cases were themselves exposed to higher levels of radiation (refer to ecological fallacy).
(b) We have not calculated any statistical measures (e.g. 95% confidence intervals or P-values) to exclude the role of chance.
(c) We have not adjusted for information bias: outdoor gamma radiation may not be a good measure of actual exposure given that many children will spend much of their time indoors.
(d) We have not adjusted for potential confounders (e.g. age, gender, population density).
(e) There is no clear dose–response relationship. However, categorizing the gamma radiation by quartile is likely to make this more difficult to detect. In reality, the lower three quartiles had smaller ranges of exposure than the fourth quartile, which may partially explain some of the similarities in risk between the lower quartiles.

Cross-sectional studies   7

Overview

Cross-sectional studies measure the frequency of outcomes and/or exposures at one point in time. The cross-sectional design can investigate large numbers of study subjects relatively rapidly. However, because the outcome and exposure are measured simultaneously, it is often difficult to know whether the exposure preceded the outcome, making it difficult to infer causality. This chapter reviews the characteristics, advantages and limitations of the cross-sectional study design for analytical epidemiology.

Learning objectives

When you have completed this chapter you should be able to:

- describe the basic uses, strengths and limitations of cross-sectional studies
- discuss potential sources of bias in cross-sectional studies
- recognize the basic analytical approaches used in cross-sectional studies.

What defines a cross-sectional study?

In a cross-sectional study, data on outcomes and/or exposures are collected on each study participant at one point in time. Cross-sectional studies have the main advantage of being relatively quick and easy to perform. They are better for measuring the frequency of chronic outcomes as they include *prevalent* rather than incident cases. Those with acute outcomes may die or resolve their symptoms before detection by cross-sectional survey.

Cross-sectional surveys provide a snapshot of a population's current health status, which can be used in the planning of health services or the determination of health practices. Repeated studies can be used to determine changes in exposure and outcome frequency over time. They therefore form a core part of routine monitoring (see Chapter 12).

Study design

The cross-sectional survey design is often used in *descriptive* epidemiological studies to estimate the frequency of outcomes *or* exposures without the intention of investigating causal associations. They may be referred to as 'prevalence surveys', as they collect data on existing (prevalent) cases of an outcome, and may be used to provide baseline descriptive data for other types of analytical studies.

An *analytical* cross-sectional study collects data on both *outcome and exposure at the same time-point* for a given study subject. Cross-sectional studies can be used to test hypotheses of association where the exposure status does not change over time (e.g. blood group antigens). However, it is often not possible to know whether the exposure preceded the outcome, and some outcomes have long latent periods, making it difficult to infer causality. For example, the time between exposure to HIV and onset of AIDS can be more than 10 years. Therefore, a cross-sectional study would not have been appropriate to investigate an association between HIV infection and AIDS prevalence in the early days of the AIDS epidemic. For this reason, cross-sectional studies are generally used for generating research hypotheses and for health service planning and monitoring, rather than for establishing causal links.

Sampling

A representative sample of the population must be selected using the methods of random selection and sample size calculation discussed in Chapter 5. In a cross-sectional study, there is no loss to follow-up, though there may be some non-response. Interviewers may include errors when filling-in questionnaires, although these can be considerably reduced by appropriate questionnaire design and training. Respondents may refuse to answer particular questions, for example, on income-level or sexual behaviours. Even clinical measures may suffer losses, for example, when taking finger-prick samples from infants to measure haemoglobin, some infants may not release sufficient blood. Many of these issues can be highlighted with a **pilot-study**, pre-testing data collection and data entry methods. However, if there is still potential for non-reponse in either the outcome or exposure of interest, the sample size should be increased to allow for this. A larger sample size will increase the statistical power and precision of the estimated frequency or association, though this may also increase the time and cost of the study.

Data collection

Cross-sectional studies may collect information using a combination of questionnaires and diagnostic tests. They allow for collection of data on many variables, and are ideal for collecting data on potential confounders for use at the analytical stage. Although data in a cross-sectional study are collected at one time-point, the measures collected may be current (e.g. blood pressure, current symptoms) or past (e.g. vaccination history, previous smoking practices).

To measure prevalence, it is important that survey questions are sufficiently specific. Asking 'Did your child have fever in the last 24 hours?' will provide an estimate of the point prevalence of (current) fever. Asking 'Has your child had fever during the last two weeks?' will record fever episodes that started prior to two weeks and continued into it, as well as episodes that started during the two-week period of interest. Surveys that relate to the prevalence of an outcome during a period of time in the past will estimate **period prevalence**. While period prevalence may increase case detection and there-fore reduce the necessary sample size, questions about past experience may also increase the possibility of *recall bias*.

Measurement of current exposure in a cross-sectional survey is appropriate when the exposure is constant (e.g. genetic markers), and will be unaffected by the outcome or potential confounders. However, some exposures may change over time, particularly in response to the outcome. For example, people with colon cancer may adapt the foods they eat to reduce discomfort, so current diet would not be a reasonable proxy for previous diet as a risk factor. Self-reported history may suffer from recall bias. Therefore, measures of past exposure from routine data (e.g. health records), or more memorable exposures (e.g. occupation, previous smoking habits), are more appropriate.

Questions need to be appropriately designed and tested to improve response rates. A question that is unclear, or that the respondent may be embarrassed to answer, can result in non-responder bias (a form of information bias). Choosing appropriate methods for the topic of investigation (interview vs. self-completed questionnaire), ensuring anonymity, and careful wording and pre-testing of questions should reduce such error.

Analysis

In an analytical cross-sectional study, the appropriate measure of association is the *prevalence ratio*. This is the ratio of the prevalence of the outcome in those exposed divided by the prevalence in those unexposed. However, when the outcome is rare (i.e. the prevalence is low), the prevalence ratio is approximately the same as the odds ratio (see Chapter 3 – Comparability of measures of association on p. 31). This is useful, because it means that we can use logistic regression models to analyse cross-sectional studies, adjusting for several potential confounders, and report results using odds ratios.

Interpretation

The results of analytical cross-sectional studies need to be interpreted with caution, because both outcome and exposure are measured simultaneously and it may not be possible to know which preceded the other. In the example of colon cancer and diet, investigating current diet as a risk factor would lead to **reverse causality**, where the exposure is actually a consequence of the outcome.

Activity 7.1

Many intervention studies have shown that mosquito nets treated with insecticide can reduce illness and mortality from malaria in young children in Africa. Investigators carried out a cross-sectional study of randomly selected children under two years of age in 18 villages in Tanzania at the beginning of a marketing campaign to promote the use of insecticide-treated nets (ITNs) (Abdulla et al. 2001). They collected data on net ownership and other factors by interviewing the mothers of young children using a questionnaire. They took blood samples from the children to test whether they were infected with malaria parasites and if they were anaemic (haemoglobin < 8g/dl) as a result. Two further cross-sectional surveys, each with a different random sample of children, were conducted over the next 2 years. Table 7.1 combines selected results from the three surveys combined.

1 What type of cross-sectional study is this?
2 Describe the results of the study shown in Table 7.1 and determine whether you can calculate the effect of net ownership on the proportion of children with malaria parasites from this table.

Table 7.1 Numbers (%) of children from three cross-sectional surveys, 1997–1999

	Year of survey		
	1997	1998	1999
Number of children eligible	325	330	330
Number of children analysed	240	269	239
Reported net ownership (%)			
no net	100 (42)	49 (18)	40 (17)
untreated net	116 (48)	64 (24)	53 (22)
ITN	24 (10)	156 (58)	146 (61)
Number (%) of children			
with anaemia (haemoglobin <8 g/dl)	118 (49)	83 (31)	62 (26)
with malaria parasites	151 (63)	126 (47)	90 (38)

Source: Abdullah et al. (2001).

Table 7.2 shows numbers of children with anaemia and malaria parasites according to net ownership for all three surveys combined.

Table 7.2 Effect of net ownership on the prevalence of anaemia and malaria parasites

	Number (%) of children		
	with anaemia	with malaria parasites	Total
Net ownership			
no net	103 (54%)	132 (70%)	189
untreated net	90 (39%)	115 (49%)	233
ITN	70 (21%)	120 (37%)	326
Total	263	367	

Source: Abdullah et al. (2001).

3 What is the prevalence ratio for anaemia of the effect of owning an ITN compared with no net?

4 What is the prevalence ratio for malaria parasites of the effect of *not* owning a net, whether ITN or untreated? Hint: Construct a 2×2 table of each outcome and exposure variable, and convert the exposure into two categories (i.e. net versus no net; ITN versus no ITN), as indicated for each question.

Activity 7.2

A survey of adolescents aged 12–16 years was undertaken in Goa, India, using a development and well-being assessment to diagnose the presence of mental disorders (Pillai et al. 2008). Structured interviews were also conducted to assess risk factors, including family relations in the previous 12 months. Eligible individuals were identified through health centre family registers and a door-to-door survey. Of 2,648 eligible adolescents, 358 were absent from home on three visits by the researcher, 85 had migrated, 187 did not consent to participate and 6 did not complete the assessment. Of the 2,048 analysed, 37 were diagnosed as having a mental disorder. Selected results of multiple logistic regression analyses are shown in Table 7.3.

Table 7.3 Selected factors associated with the presence of a mental disorder in adolescents (n = 2048)

Risk factor	Odds ratio (95% CI)	P-value
Physical/verbal abuse from parents:		0.02
Never/rarely	1.00	
Occasionally	1.50 (0.6, 3.7)	
Often	2.90 (1.3, 6.8)	
Perceived family support:		0.01
Rarely	1.00	
Sometimes	0.18 (0.1, 0.7)	
Often	0.15 (0.04, 0.5)	
Always	0.16 (0.1, 0.5)	

Source: Pillai (2008).

> 1 What are the two hypotheses being tested in Table 7.3? (Note, the *reference* or unexposed group is that with an odds ratio of 1.00.)
> 2 Interpret the results in Table 7.3, with reference to the trends in odds ratios, 95% confidence intervals and *P*-values.
> 3 What potential sources of bias can you identify from the information given, and how might these affect interpretation of the results?

Conclusion

In this chapter you have reviewed the key features, advantages and disadvantages of cross-sectional studies. This study design is a relatively cheap and cost-effective way to collect descriptive epidemiological data. In analytical epidemiology, cross-sectional studies may suffer from bias, confounding, and issues of reverse causality if the exposure is not constant. This is therefore not the design of choice for inferring causality.

References

Abdulla S, Schellenberg JA, Nathan R, et al. (2001) Impact on malaria morbidity of a programme supplying insecticide treated nets in children aged under 2 years in Tanzania: community cross-sectional study. *British Medical Journal* 322: 270–3.
Pillai A, Patel V, Cardozo P, et al. (2008) Non-traditional lifestyles and prevalence of mental disorders in adolescents in Goa, India. *British Journal of Psychiatry* 192: 45–51.

Feedback on activities

Activity 7.1

1 This is an analytical cross-sectional study, because the investigators are interested in the effect that the preventive measure of using insecticide-treated nets (ITNs) will have on the prevalence of malaria in children.

2 The results in Table 7.1 suggest that ownership of ITNs increases over the period of the study, while the number of households with no nets or untreated nets, and the proportion of children with anaemia or malaria parasites, decreases over the course of the study. However, from Table 7.1 it is not possible to calculate the effect of net ownership on the proportion of children with malaria, because we have not been given the numbers of children with either anaemia or malaria parasites in each of the net ownership categories.

3 To calculate the prevalence ratio for anaemia of the effect of ITNs compared with no net ownership, your 2×2 table should look like Table 7.4, with appropriate labelling.

Table 7.4 ITN ownership among children with and without anaemia

| | Number of children | | |
	Anaemia	No anaemia	Total
ITN	70	256	326
No net	103	86	189
Total	173	342	515

Source: Adapted from Bailey et al. (2005).

To compare the prevalence of anaemia in the two exposure groups:
Prevalence of anaemia in those with ITNs = 70 ÷ 326 = 0.215 or 21.5%.
Prevalence of anaemia in those without nets = 103 ÷ 189 = 0.545 or 54.5%.
Therefore the prevalence ratio is 0.215 ÷ 0.545 = 0.394 or 39.4%.

A prevalence ratio of 0.39 indicates that children in households with ITNs have 39% the risk of anaemia as those in households without nets. This is the same as saying that children with ITNs have 61% (1 − 0.394 = 0.606) lower prevalence of anaemia than those without nets.

4 To calculate the prevalence ratio for malaria parasites of the effect of *no* net ownership compared with *any* net ownership, your 2×2 table should look like Table 7.5.

Table 7.5 Net ownership among children with and without malaria parasites

| | Number of children | | |
	with parasites	without parasites	Total
No net	132	57	189
Net	235	324	559
Total	367	381	748

Source: Adapted from Bailey et al. (2005).

To compare the prevalence of malaria parasites in the two exposure groups:
Prevalence of parasites in those without nets = 132 ÷ 189 = 0.698 or 69.8%.
Prevalence of parasites in those with nets = 235 ÷ 559 = 0.420 or 42.0%.
Therefore the prevalence ratio is 0.698 ÷ 0.420 = 1.66, indicating that children in households without nets have a 66% higher prevalence of parasites than those with nets.

Activity 7.2

1 Hypothesis 1: 'The prevalence of mental disorder in adolescents in this population *increases* with more frequent physical or verbal abuse from parents.' OR 'Prevalence is *greater* among adolescents exposed to occasional or frequent physical/verbal abuse from parents than those exposed to no or rare physical/verbal abuse from parents.'

Hypothesis 2: 'The prevalence of mental disorder in adolescents in this population *decreases* with more frequent family support.' OR 'Prevalence is *lower* in adolescents who receive support from their family (sometimes/often/always) than in those rarely supported by their family.'

2 In Table 7.3, the odds ratio of mental disorders appears to increase with increasing frequency of physical/verbal abuse from parents. The overall P-value of 0.02, means that there is less than a 2% chance that this association would be observed if it did not truly exist. The 95% confidence interval for occasional abuse from parents is 0.6 – 3.7 which includes the value 1.00, therefore individuals in this category are not at a significantly increased risk of mental disorder than those in the never/rarely category. However, the 95% confidence interval for the 'often' category is 1.3 – 6.8, which does not include 1.00, indicating that adolescents 'often' exposed to abuse from parents have almost three times (odds ratio = 2.90), greater odds of mental disorder than those 'never/rarely' exposed to abuse from parents.

The odds ratio of mental disorders is much lower in adolescents who reported family support 'sometimes', 'often' or 'always', compared to those who reported family support 'rarely'. The overall P-value of 0.01 means there is less than a 1% chance that this association would be observed if it did not truly exist. However, there does not appear to be much of a trend as all categories had similar odds ratios (0.18, 0.15, 0.16), and their 95% confidence intervals overlapped with each other. This suggests that the measure of level of family support did not discriminate well between the different categories. All three categories of adolescents who reported some family support had 95% confidence intervals that did not include 1.0, indicating that they were all significantly different from those who reported 'rarely' receiving family support. In summary, adolescents reporting some family support had between 82–85% lower odds of suffering from a mental disorder.

3 There is likely to be *selection bias*. The 358 absent adolescents, 187 who refused to consent, and 6 who did not complete assessment, may have been different from the individuals analysed in relation to outcome or exposures. As this totals 20% of those eligible, such potential bias in the estimate of effect makes it difficult to generalize the results to the target population.

There is likely to be *information bias*, as exposures were all self-reported. The investigators developed structured interviews that had previously been tested elsewhere, and also interviewed a sibling for 36% of participants. Given the high levels of stigma associated with the topic, there may have been under-reporting of abuse by parents, which may be non-differential and lead to an underestimate of the strength of the association.

There may also be *reverse causality*, if individuals with mental disorders have different perceptions of their interactions and are, for example, more prone to perceiving abuse by parents or lack of family support.

8 Cohort studies

Overview

Cohort studies measure the exposures of interest and then follow up study participants over time to measure the *incidence* of the outcome of interest. Cohort studies are a type of natural experiment because defined groups are followed, as they would be in an intervention trial, although the investigator's job is purely to observe and not to intervene. This is one of the best analytical designs as the definition of exposure prior to outcome may reduce problems of selection and participant bias. In this chapter you will review the characteristics, advantages and limitations of the cohort study design for analytical epidemiology.

Learning objectives

When you have completed this chapter you should be able to:

- describe the uses, strengths and limitations of cohort studies
- discuss the potential sources of bias in cohort studies
- recognize the basic analytical approaches commonly used.

What defines a cohort study?

Epidemiologists use the term *cohort* to describe a group of individuals who share a common characteristic, and are followed up to measure the *incidence* of an outcome. A cohort may be a group of workers from a factory, a group of children who were born in the same year, or a group of individuals at risk of a particular outcome. The exposures of interest are recorded at the start of the study, and may be updated during the study. Cohort studies are therefore more likely than other observational study designs to meet the temporality criterion for causality (see Chapter 4).

Cohort studies are most often used when the outcome of interest is common, as a rare outcome would require too large a sample size. They may also be used to study relatively *rare exposures* by careful selection of participants on the basis of their exposure. The incidence of an outcome in an exposed cohort is compared with that in an unexposed cohort to see whether the exposure results in any observable difference.

Cohort studies enable us to study a wide range of outcomes that may be associated with a single exposure of interest. Even an outcome that was not anticipated at the start of the study may be included in data collection during the course of the study. This is especially useful when dealing with the introduction of new exposures whose health risks are undefined (e.g. mobile phone use, wireless technologies).

The main disadvantages of cohort studies are: (a) the large number of participants required; (b) the cost of data collection for active **follow-up** (e.g. health evaluations, quality-of-life questionnaires) versus passive follow-up (e.g. death or cancer notifications); and (c) the length of the study, as some prospective cohort studies may take decades to complete.

Study design

The cohort design can be used in *descriptive* studies to provide baseline data, and for routine monitoring (see Chapter 12). The observational nature of the design may sometimes raise ethical conflicts when dealing with severe and potentially fatal outcomes, as any interference by the investigator can have an impact on the outcomes being measured.

Analytical cohort studies (also known as *incidence studies, longitudinal studies, or follow-up studies*) can be prospective or retrospective. However, both types define the cohort on the basis of *exposure* and not outcome status. It can be helpful to present the flow of numbers of study participants when describing a cohort study (see Figure 8.1).

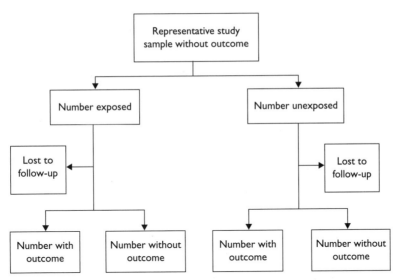

Figure 8.1 Flow-chart of numbers of participants recruited, numbers categorized as exposed or unexposed, numbers lost-to-follow-up in each category, and numbers with and without the outcome in each exposure category at the end of the study

Source: Ilona Carneiro.

Prospective cohorts identify participants and then follow them over time until they either acquire the outcome of interest or the time limit for the study has been reached. The main feature of prospective cohort studies is that data on exposures are collected *before* data on the outcome. Study participants must be free of the outcome of interest at the start of the study. For example, if the outcome is having cancer, it is important to ensure that all participants are cancer-free at the start of the study. Prospective cohorts have a major advantage over other study types in determining whether an exposure might be causally associated with the outcome, since we can be fairly sure in which order the exposure and outcome occurred and outcome status cannot affect the classification of exposure status.

Retrospective cohorts use pre-existing data on exposures and outcomes – for example, from medical or occupational records – and therefore do not need to follow individuals over time since all the information is already available. These are usually quicker and cheaper to carry out than prospective studies, particularly for diseases or events that may take decades to develop (e.g. cancer). However, routine data may be poorly collected (e.g. inaccurate, missing data), may not provide necessary information on other important risk factors or confounders, and may be liable to changes in defini- tions and coding systems over time.

A cohort study may combine both retrospective and prospective data. For example, a study may identify a cohort of children aged 2 years old and follow them for a year to measure the incidence of vaccine preventable diseases, while using vaccination records that pre-date the start of the study to provide information on prior exposures.

Sampling

Selection of the study population usually depends on whether the exposure of interest is common or rare. If the exposure is common, we can select the study population before classifying each individual as exposed or unexposed, for example, a random sample of the general population. Information on exposure can then be collected as the individuals are followed up, and the original selection of the cohort purely depends on the group being disease-free at the start of the study.

Alternatively, the study population could be selected from a particular occupation group (e.g. nurses, government workers, or mine workers) or by place of work (e.g. factory, other large institution). This is known as a *workforce* or *occupational cohort* and has the advantage of higher participation and higher level of follow-up than general population cohorts. It usually does not matter that the workforce cohort is not representative of the general population, as long as the exposed and unexposed groups are comparable within the cohort.

If the exposure is rare, the study sample can be selected on the basis of exposure to make sure that enough exposed people are included to make the study viable. For example, if the exposure of interest is contact with industrial chemicals, then workers at a particular factory, known to handle chemicals as part of their job, can be chosen as the exposure group. The comparison group would then be selected from workers at the same factory who did not work with those chemicals. This is known as an *internal comparison group*. However, if all workers at the factory had some degree of exposure, we would need to select a comparison group from another population, possibly another type of factory, to ensure that the comparison group only differed in terms of their exposure and not in terms of other factors. This would be an *external comparison group*, and would be chosen from another workforce to avoid the *healthy worker effect* (a form of *selection bias* that tends to underestimate excess risk associated with an occupation by comparing with the general population, which includes people too sick to work).

The sample size is related to the amount of time that participants are followed up. For example, if the sample size for a study is calculated as 1,000 person years at risk, the study could follow-up 1,000 people for one year, or 500 people for two years, or 250 people for four years. However, a longer follow-up time implies a greater likelihood of loss of contact with participants. This 'loss to follow-up' needs to be accounted for by increasing the initial sample size to cover expected losses. For example, if we expect we may lose contact with 10% of participants over the course of a two-year study, the number of participants recruited to the study should be 10% greater than the calculated sample size.

Data collection

For a retrospective study, data are usually collected from routine sources, such as patient hospital records, workplace personnel records or death notifications. For a prospective cohort study, data on exposures can be collected similarly to a cross-sectional study. This includes interviewing participants, consulting medical records, taking biological samples, or using other forms of routine data. Exposures that are not going to change during the study, such as date of birth, sex, birthweight, adult height, blood type and genetic factors, are collected when participants enter the study. Exposures that may change, such as blood pressure, physical activity, smoking, or disease status, are collected by re-assessing individuals in the cohort at predefined time-points during the study, or sometimes from medical records as and when they occur. If data on the exposure are detailed, there may be an opportunity to study dose–response relationships between exposure and outcome. Detailed information on confounding factors can also be collected, allowing investigators to control for them in the analysis. Outcomes may be collected through periodic health examinations or health outcome questionnaires to members of the cohort.

The length of follow-up needed for a sufficient proportion of the participants to have acquired an outcome may be many years (even decades for more rare outcomes). This can make cohort studies expensive and time-consuming to conduct, although occupational cohorts are easier and cheaper to follow up where record-keeping systems on employees already exist.

Analysis

If the cohort study is descriptive, we can measure the frequency of outcome as a *risk* or a *rate*. If the follow-up times for all participants are similar, then we can use the risk. If the follow-up times differ between participants, and person-time at risk is known, then a rate would be more appropriate.

In an analytical cohort study the appropriate measure of epidemiological association is the *risk ratio* or *rate ratio*, depending on the frequency measure used. Measures of impact such as *attributable risk, attributable fraction, population attributable risk* and *population attributable fraction* can also be calculated (see Chapter 3). Using regression models allows us to adjust for the effect of potential confounders (see Chapter 5).

If data are being compared between two cohorts that do not have the same demographic structure (e.g. age, sex), the result may be confounded by these other factors. This may occur when comparing males and females, two cohorts selected from different populations, or the study cohort with the general population. In these cases it is necessary to standardize the incidence using a standard population structure (see Chapter 6).

Time-series analysis

As some exposures may vary over time, it is important that any changes in exposure status are recorded and updated. A more complex statistical technique called *time-series analysis* can be used to take account of changes in exposure, timing of outcome and for more detailed changes in person-time at risk (e.g. temporary movement out of the study area). Results of such analyses may be presented graphically as a survival curve or a failure curve. Such graphs can be used for any outcome, where failure represents acquisition of the outcome (e.g. incidence of cancer) and survival represents the lack of outcome (e.g. those *not* rejecting an organ after a transplant operation).

Figure 8.2 shows a child survival curve from a cohort study in rural Bangladesh, comparing those whose mother had died before the child's tenth birthday to those whose mother had not. The distance between the two lines provides a graphical representation of the relative effect of maternal mortality and enables us to see how the effect changes over time (in this case, by age of the child).

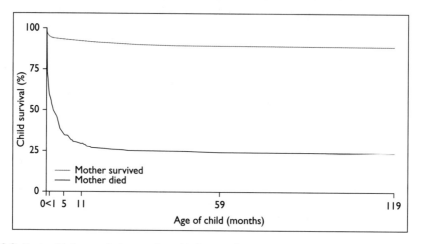

Figure 8.2 Kaplan-Meier survival curve from birth according to survival status of mother
Source: Ronsmans et al. (2010).

Interpretation

As with other analytical studies, any observed association between exposure and out-come may be affected by *chance, bias and confounding* and consideration needs to be given to how these may have affected the results.

Selection bias may occur if the selected cohort participants are not representative of the target population. High rates of *loss to follow-up* or differences in the loss to follow-up between exposure groups can also lead to selection bias. For example, if long-term follow-up is conducted by a self-completed questionnaire, participants may be less likely to respond due to death, disability, moving into a nursing home, etc. Similarly, if cohorts have been selected according to their exposure status, it is important that the exposed and unexposed cohorts are not different with respect to other factors that have not been measured. For example, if an occupational cohort of asbestos removal workers were compared with the general population, a finding of increased risk of lung cancer would not provide useful information, as we could not eliminate the occupation. However, by comparing within the cohort, we can investigate the risks associated with type of respirator used and number of exposure hours, for example, to provide recommendations for appropriate occupation regulations.

Observer bias may occur if knowledge of exposure status affects classification of outcome status, or in retrospective cohorts if knowledge of the outcome status affects classification of exposure status. This may lead to *systematic misclassification bias* (see Chapter 4).

Activity 8.1

In 1951, a prospective cohort study was initiated to investigate the relationship between smoking and mortality among British doctors, particularly mortality due to lung cancer (Doll and Peto 1976; Doll et al. 1980). This is an important study, which ultimately followed up participants for 50 years (Doll et al. 2004).

In 1951, a questionnaire on smoking habits was sent to 49,913 male and 10,323 female doctors registered with the British General Medical Council; 34,440 male doctors and 6,194 female doctors gave sufficient information to classify their smoking status. The vital status of these doctors was followed up from the records of the Registrar General's Office, the British Medical Council and the British Medical Association. The causes of death of 10,072 male and 1,094 female doctors who had died during the first 20 and 22 years of follow-up respectively were ascertained from death certificates. The rate of death from lung cancer among smokers was compared to that among non-smokers.

1. Discuss the potential sources of bias in this study.
2. Identify what information on smoking you would collect to classify smoking exposure status.
3. Age-adjusted lung cancer death rates per 100,000 persons per year among smokers and non-smokers in male and female doctors are given in Table 8.1. Calculate appropriate epidemiological measures of association between smoking and lung cancer and discuss the result, especially the differences between males and females.

Table 8.1 Lung cancer death rates per 100,000 person-years by gender and smoking status

Gender	Lung cancer death rates per 100,000 persons per year			
	Non-smokers	Smoking 1–14 cigarettes/day	Smoking 15–24 cigarettes/day	Smoking 25+ cigarettes/day
Male	10	78	127	251
Female	7	9	45	208

Source: Bailey et al. (2005), using data from Doll and Peto (1976) and Doll et al. (1980).

Activity 8.2

A study of the effect of HIV infection on the incidence of pulmonary tuberculosis (TB) was undertaken in the year 2000. Investigators analysed data from personnel and medical records between 1991–1997 on miners working at four gold mines in South Africa (Sonnenberg et al. 2005). Using unique employee numbers, a confidential database of HIV results from tests performed with consent was linked to data on the incidence of first episode of pulmonary TB from annual chest-radiograph screening.

Table 8.2 Incidence of pulmonary tuberculosis (TB) by HIV status and age

Category	Person-years at risk	Pulmonary TB cases	Incidence per 100 person-years at risk	Rate ratio
HIV negative miners	36,020	289		1.00
HIV positive miners	15,561	451		3.61
Age:				
<30 years	15,483	103	0.67	
30–39 years	24,645	387	1.57	
40–49 years	8,670	176	2.03	
≥ 50 years	2,783	74	2.66	

Source: Sonnenberg et al. (2005).

1 What type of study design is this? Be as specific as you can.
2 Calculate the missing values in Table 8.2 for:
   (a) the incidence of pulmonary TB according to HIV infection status.
   (b) the incidence rate ratio for pulmonary TB by age group.
3 The 95% confidence interval (CI) for the rate ratio of pulmonary TB with HIV infection is 3.12–4.19. How would you interpret this result?
4 The rate ratio of pulmonary TB by HIV infection status after adjusting for the effect of age and calendar period of the study was 2.90 (95% CI: 2.48–3.38). From this information and the results in Table 8.2, do you think that age is a confounder in the association between HIV and pulmonary TB?

Conclusion

In this chapter, you have reviewed the key features, advantages and disadvantages of cohort studies. As exposure to a risk factor is usually determined before outcome in cohort studies, this design enables us to assess temporality when inferring causality. Biases can be minimized through appropriate study design and data on confounding factors can be collected for adjustment during analysis, making this the most appropriate observational study design for investigating epidemiological associations.

References

Doll R, Gray R, Hafner B and Peto R (1980) Mortality in relation to smoking: 22 years' observations on female British doctors. *British Medical Journal* 280: 967–71.

Doll R and Peto R (1976) Mortality in relation to smoking: 20 years' observations on male British doctors. *British Medical Journal* 2: 1525–36.

Doll R, Peto R, Boreham J and Sutherland I (2004) Mortality in relation to smoking: 50 years' observations on male British doctors. *British Medical Journal* 328: 1519.

Ronsmans C, Chowdhury ME, Dasgupta SK, Ahmed A and Koblinsky M (2010) Effect of parent's death on child survival in rural Bangladesh: a cohort study. *Lancet* 375: 2024–31.

Sonnenberg P, Glynn JR, Fielding K, et al. (2005) How soon after infection with HIV does the risk of tuberculosis start to increase? A retrospective cohort study in South African gold miners. *Journal of Infectious Disease* 191: 150–8.

Feedback on activities

Activity 8.1

1 This is effectively an occupational cohort. Therefore, actual estimates from the study may not be directly extrapolated to the general population, because of the *healthy worker effect*. Doctors are also likely to have had better access to good medical care than the general population.

   There may be some *selection bias*. First, only 69% (34,400/49,913) of eligible male doctors and 60% (6,194/10,323) eligible female doctors gave sufficient information to be included in the cohort. Those who did not respond, or gave incomplete information may have been different from those who did respond in a way that may also have affected their exposure or risk of outcome.

   Second, it is unlikely that investigators were able to follow up all subjects for the full period, due to migration or loss of records (i.e. *loss to follow-up*). However, in this study, where the sample size is large and the routine reporting systems are robust, this is unlikely to have greatly affected the result.

   There may have been some *information bias*. First, if some doctors gave inaccurate information regarding their smoking habits, this could have resulted in misclassification of exposure to smoking. At the time of classification of exposure to smoking in 1951, the association with lung cancer was not commonly known. Some case-control studies had indicated an association, and some doctors may have been aware of this, but they would not have known their own future risk of lung cancer. Therefore, any such responder bias would likely result in *non-differential misclassification* and underestimate the strength of the association.

   Second, there could have been *observer bias* if lung cancer was more frequently diagnosed or certified as the cause of death among smokers than among non-smokers. However, this is unlikely since doctors would be likely to have access to good medical care and lung cancer can be diagnosed accurately using various radiographic and histological investigations. In addition, the cause of death was obtained from death certificates and not diagnosed by study investigators.

2 A simple categorization could be to classify individuals as current smokers, former smokers or lifelong non-smokers. However, the effect of smoking may vary by the age doctors started to smoke, age of stopping smoking for former smokers, type of smoke (i.e. cigarette, cigar, pipe), and a dose effect may be investigated by quantifying the amount smoked (i.e. number of cigarettes per day, inhalation of smoke, second-hand smoke). Information on all these variables should be collected.

3 As rates are given in Table 8.1, the appropriate measure of association is the incidence rate ratio of lung cancer deaths among different categories of smokers for males and females. It would be most appropriate to use the death rate in non-smokers as the reference 'unexposed' category.

   The rate ratio for lung cancer among males smoking 1–14 cigarettes per day compared with male non-smokers is calculated as follows (you may wish to refer to Chapter 3):

$$\text{Incidence rate ratio} = \frac{78}{10} = 7.8$$

Similarly, the rate ratio for lung cancer among females smoking 25+ cigarettes per day compared with female non-smokers is calculated as follows:

$$\text{Incidence rate ratio} = \frac{208}{7} = 29.7$$

You should have calculated the remaining incidence rate ratios from Table 8.1 as shown in Table 8.3. Note, the rate ratio for the reference category is always 1.00.

Table 8.3 Incidence rate ratios for lung cancer death by gender and smoking status

Gender	Lung cancer death rates per 100,000 persons per year			
	Non-smokers	Smoking 1–14 cigarettes/day	Smoking 15–24 cigarettes/day	Smoking 25+ cigarettes/day
Male	1	7.8	12.7	25.1
Female	1	1.3	6.4	29.7

Source: Bailey et al. (2005).

The rate ratio for lung cancer death increased with the quantity smoked among both male and female doctors. This dose–response effect lends support to a causal association between smoking and lung cancer.

The rate ratio in men smoking 1–14 and 15–24 cigarettes per day is much higher than in women. In those smoking 25 or more cigarettes per day, the rate ratio in men is marginally less than that in women. Does this mean that the effect of low levels of smoking is higher among men than among women? Without carrying out statistical tests, we cannot know whether these rate ratios are significantly different, but the study had a large sample size and the magnitude of difference is high, so it is unlikely to be due to *chance*. However, number of cigarettes smoked is unlikely to be a sufficiently good estimate of overall exposure to tobacco, which will also be affected by other factors such as the age of starting smoking (which was later among women than men in this cohort), and inhalation (more men than women in this cohort reported inhaling). These other factors modify the effect of number of cigarettes smoked on lung cancer death.

Activity 8.2

1 This is a *retrospective occupational cohort* study. Retrospective, because data on both exposure and outcome are taken from routine data collected prior to the analysis. Occupational, because all study participants share the same occupation, and employee records were used to obtain data. Cohort, because the outcome frequency measure is incidence.

2 The completed table should look like Table 8.4.
   (a) The incidence rate is calculated as the number of new (incident) TB cases divided by the person-time at risk for each category. For example, for HIV negative miners, the incidence is 289 ÷ 36,020 = 0.0080 cases per person-year at risk, or 0.8 cases per 100 person-years at risk.

Table 8.4 Incidence of tuberculosis (TB) by HIV status and age

Category	Person-years at risk	TB cases	Incidence per 100 person-years at risk	Rate ratio
HIV negative miners	36,020	289	0.80	1.00
HIV positive miners	15,561	451	2.90	3.61
Age:				
<30 years	15,483	103	0.67	1.00
30–39 years	24,645	387	1.57	2.34
40–49 years	8,670	176	2.03	3.03
≥ 50 years	2,783	74	2.66	3.97

Source: Ilona Carneiro, using data from Sonnenberg et al. (2005).

(b) The incidence rate ratio is calculated as the rate in the exposed group divided by the rate in the unexposed group. For example, the rate ratio of TB for age 30–39 years compared with <30 years is 1.57 ÷ 0.67 = 2.34. You may have used a different reference category, which would also be correct as long as the rate ratio for the reference category is listed as 1.00.

3 A rate ratio of 3.61 indicates that the risk of pulmonary TB in this cohort is more than three times greater in miners with HIV infection than in those without HIV. This is a statistically significant result with less than 5% probability that it is due to chance, as the 95% confidence interval does not include the value 1.00. We can be 95% certain that the true estimate of association between HIV and pulmonary TB in this mining population is between 3.12 and 4.19.

4 There is a clear association between age and the incidence of pulmonary TB, as the rate ratio increases with age, and all estimates are statistically significant. It is also possible that age is associated with HIV infection status, although we do not have that information. The change in rate ratio after adjusting for age and study period suggests that the initial estimate of association between pulmonary TB and HIV may be partly explained by the effects of age and study period. This suggests that age may be a confounder in the association between pulmonary TB and HIV infection. However, we would need to know the association between age and HIV, and the rate ratio of pulmonary TB by HIV infection adjusted *only* for age group, to be sure.

9 Case-control studies

Overview

Case-control studies take the opposite approach to cohort studies, by identifying those with and without the outcome, and then determining their previous exposure to potential risk factors. This approach is especially useful for rare outcomes, as well as being cheaper and faster than cohort studies, as the sample size can be smaller and there is no need for lengthy follow-up. However, with this design it is impossible to estimate the frequency of an outcome and it is more difficult to avoid bias. In this chapter you will review the characteristics, advantages and limitations of the case-control study design for analytical epidemiology.

Learning objectives

When you have completed this chapter you should be able to:

- describe the uses, strengths and limitations of case-control studies
- discuss potential sources of bias in case-control studies
- recognize the basic analytical approaches used in case-control studies.

What defines a case-control study?

In case-control studies, the study groups are defined by *outcome* and not by exposure. Groups are selected on the basis of whether they do (**cases**) or do not (**controls**) have the outcome under study at the *beginning* of the study. The cases are then compared with controls to assess whether they are different in terms of their previous exposure to particular risk factors. It is therefore impossible to estimate the frequency (i.e. prevalence, risk, odds or incidence rate) of the outcome in the target population.

Advantages and disadvantages

Case-control studies were first developed in the early 1950s to avoid some of the disadvantages of cohort studies. One of the advantages of case-control studies is that they can be used to study rare outcomes. As participants are selected according to their outcome status, it is possible to recruit the minimum number of cases and controls required before the study begins. A cohort study requires follow-up of prohibitively large numbers of individuals to ensure that enough participants develop a rare outcome.

The case-control design is also useful when a rapid result is required, as with outbreak investigations, or with the appearance of a new syndrome (e.g. AIDS). Case-control studies can also be more efficient than cohort studies when there is a long period of time between the exposure and outcome (latency period), as for chronic diseases such as cancer or AIDS. As the exposure is classified after the outcome, it is also possible to investigate the association with multiple exposures.

One of the problems with case-control studies is that both exposure and outcome have occurred by the time the patient is recruited into the study, making the design susceptible to selection and information bias.

Genetic epidemiology

Case-control studies are especially useful in genetic epidemiology (Khoury and Beaty 1994), where the interaction between genetic and environmental factors is investigated, because genes do not change with time. The sequencing of the human genome has led to the search for disease susceptibility genes, and the case-control design enables investigation of several genetic markers (and potentially the whole genome) in the same study. In addition, genetic mutations are rare, requiring clinical and laboratory tests that would be prohibitively expensive in a cohort study. However, when studying associations within families, this may not be an appropriate design because of the risk of *overmatching* (see below). Note that gender, ethnicity and other forms of population structuring are likely to be confounders in studies of genetic traits and outcomes.

Study design

One way to reduce confounding in the study design is to identify controls with the same characteristics as the cases – this is known as **matching**. However, matching can be more complicated and costly, and is not necessary as long as sufficient data on potential confounders are collected to enable adjustment in the analysis.

A special type of case-control design is the **nested case-control** study. In this design, cases are members of a cohort that have developed the outcome, and controls are those without the outcome. This allows us to automatically match on factors common to all cohort members. For instance, in an occupational cohort study, cases and controls will be matched on employment status simply by virtue of being in that cohort. This form of study design also means that new hypotheses can be tested more easily, since data on exposures are likely to have already been collected as part of the cohort study, which will save time and money. As data on exposures will have been collected prior to the outcome, there is less chance of recall and observer bias, and it is easier to establish the temporal condition for causality.

Sampling

As participants are selected on the basis of their outcome and will be compared by their exposure, it is important that the participants are representative of the target population in relation to the frequency of the exposure, and that the selection of cases and controls is not influenced by their exposure (*selection bias*).

The case definition must be very precise and inclusion and exclusion criteria must be clearly stated before the study is conducted to ensure that the practice of identifying cases is kept uniform throughout the study. It is necessary to consider whether both incident and prevalent cases should be included. Inclusion of prevalent cases may make it easier to generalize the study to the target population. However, prevalent cases may differ from incident cases in ways that may reduce the validity of the study. Inclusion of prevalent cases, especially for chronic outcomes, can create problems for determining exposure to certain risk factors that may change over time. This may lead to **reverse causality** where the exposure changes as a result of the outcome (e.g. diet or exercise regime).

Inclusion of prevalent cases may also lead to under-representation of more severe cases of a rapidly progressive outcome, who will die sooner after diagnosis and be less likely to be selected for the study. This in turn may affect the associations being investigated, as exposures associated with increased survival may be associated with the outcome, even though they might be protective against the development of severe disease. If the outcome is fatal, it is important to ensure that patients who have died are included to avoid selection bias.

An important consideration is the source of cases and controls. For example, if an outcome is particularly severe, it may mean that cases are only found in hospitals. If the outcome is rare or unusual, it is important to make sure that all locations of patients are identified, as patients may travel out of their local hospital catchment area to get specialist treatment, for example, at a referral hospital.

Although the recruitment process can be easier if cases are hospital-based, this makes it more difficult to identify appropriate controls. If there is some selection of who reaches hospital, then it may be appropriate to recruit controls from among other hospital patients, as long as their selection is not then biased in terms of the exposure of interest. For example, we may want to investigate risk factors for liver cirrhosis. If we suspect heavy alcohol use to be a major risk factor and select cases from hospital records, we may have problems if our hospital-based controls include a large proportion of people admitted to hospital for trauma, since people admitted for this reason are known to be more likely to be heavy users of alcohol than the general population. If all people with the outcome go to hospital, and there is no other selection process involved in the cases reaching hospital other than the outcome and the exposures under consideration, then controls can be selected from the general population.

If cases can be selected from the general population, then controls can be randomly selected from the same population with less likelihood of selection bias. Controls should meet all the criteria for cases (i.e. be as similar as possible), except for the outcome itself. For example, if the cases are men aged 40–65 years with lung cancer, the controls should be selected from men of that age group who do not have lung cancer.

Matching

Matching may be used to reduce confounding of the association between exposure and outcome, where confounders are known or highly probable. *Individual matching* identifies between one and four controls for each case, with the same age or gender. Other potential confounders, such as place of residence or ethnic group may also be used, depending on the aim of the study. Be careful not to select too many characteristics on which to match, or to select factors that might be very closely associated with exposure status. This can lead to **overmatching**, such that cases and controls do not differ sufficiently in relation to the main exposure of interest and we are unable to measure the association.

An example of overmatching comes from an early case-control study of AIDS (Moss et al. 1987), where investigators compared AIDS cases with two age-matched

homosexual male control groups. The first control was selected from the same neighbourhood as each case, while the second control was selected from those attending a
clinic for sexually transmitted infections (STIs). The study found that cases were
52 times more likely to have >100 *versus* 0–5 sexual partners in the previous year
compared with HIV-negative neighbourhood controls, but only 2.9 times more likely
when compared with HIV-negative clinic controls. This is because STIs are associated
with number of sexual partners, so clinic controls were biased towards having more
partners.

An alternative to individual matching is *frequency matching*, in which the control *group*
is selected to be similar to the case *group* regarding the matched variable. To frequency-
match by gender, for example, if our cases were 60% female, we would need to select
controls that were also 60% female.

Data collection

Case-control studies start with assessment of the outcome, so collection of information
on exposures is almost always retrospective. Exposure data can be gathered in many
different ways, including by interview (e.g. face-to-face, self-completed questionnaire),
from records (e.g. medical, employer), or from biological samples. Ideally, the researcher
collecting exposure information should not know whether the study participant is a
case or control to avoid *observer bias*.

Reporting bias is more likely in case-control studies, as knowledge of being a case (or
control) may affect what individuals remember, or how they report events or exposures. Cases may be more likely to remember events that occurred at around the time
they were diagnosed with disease or underwent a traumatic event. For example, parents of children who develop autism may be more likely than other parents to remember the date of a vaccination, if it occurred in the days preceding a change in their
child's behaviour. For this reason, it is important to use routinely collected data, or
memory guides and prompts, when collecting data on exposure.

Analysis

Case-control studies do not randomly sample the population, instead selecting individuals on the basis of their outcome status. Therefore, they cannot directly estimate
prevalence or incidence of the outcome or frequency of the exposure in the general
population. The outcome measure for a case-control study is therefore the *odds ratio
of exposure* (see Chapter 3), which is the odds of exposure in cases divided by the odds
of exposure in controls. This has the same numerical value as the odds ratio of outcome, although the interpretation is different. For example, in a case-control study
measuring the association between stress and traffic accidents, an exposure odds ratio
of 1.82 indicates that cases (individuals in a traffic accident) have 82% greater odds of
exposure to stress than controls. If the outcome is rare and the exposure is reasonably
common, this measure approximates the risk ratio.

If the study is matched, then a more complicated analysis needs to be performed to
account for matching. In this type of analysis, only the matched groups that are discord-
ant (i.e. where either the case is exposed and the control unexposed, or the case is
unexposed and the control exposed) are compared to give the odds ratio of exposure.
This is because pairs where both case and control are exposed, or both case and control

are unexposed, provide no information on differences in exposure. This can be done using conditional logistic regression.

Interpretation

Even if an association between exposure and outcome is found, the investigator still must consider whether the result could have arisen through chance, bias or confounding. As noted previously, the case-control design is especially prone to selection bias and reporting bias, because exposure is determined after outcome. Precautions should be taken to avoid *observer bias* when collecting data on exposures (e.g. blinding data collectors to the outcome status). For chronic outcomes or those with a long latent period (e.g. AIDS), there may be a possibility of *reverse causality*, when the outcome causes the exposure (e.g. change in diet) to occur before symptoms of the outcome were identified.

Activity 9.1

A review of epidemiological studies of the association between alcohol consumption and breast cancer identified 27 case-control studies, 8 cohort studies and 5 ecological studies carried out between 1977 and 1992 (Rosenberg et al. 1993).

1 Why do you think more investigators preferred the case-control study design over the other designs?

Activity 9.2

It is now well accepted that early age at menarche (first menstrual cycle), late age at menopause (end of fertility), nulliparity (never having given birth), and late age at first birth are risk factors for breast cancer in women.

A case-control study investigated the relation between alcohol and breast cancer in women. Some 160 women aged under 75 years were treated for newly diagnosed breast cancer at four hospitals. Of these women, 30 could not be interviewed because the patient refused, their consultant refused or the patient was too ill to be interviewed. The remaining 130 women were interviewed at hospital within 6 months of diagnosis by one of six interviewers. The investigators recruited 520 controls who were attending the same hospital for other conditions. The interviewers were aware of the hypothesis, and which women were cases and which were controls.

1 Why do you think that cases in the study were restricted to:
   (a) women who had been diagnosed with breast cancer in the 6 months before the interview?
   (b) women who were attending hospital?
2 If you were designing a questionnaire for this study, what information on alcohol consumption would you ask for? What other questions would you consider necessary?
3 If you were one of the study investigators, from where would you have selected your controls, and what would your inclusion and exclusion criteria have been?

4 If the investigators had matched the controls to cases, what matching variables should they have used?

5 Describe potential sources of bias in the study design.

Activity 9.3

In May 1997, a 3-year-old boy died of a respiratory illness labelled as 'avian' influenza A (H5N1). A case-control study was carried out in Hong Kong in January 1998 to identify risk factors for an outbreak of influenza A (H5N1) after 15 patients were hospitalized with the disease (Mounts et al. 1999). Two age- and gender-matched controls were identified for each case by randomly selecting a neighbouring apartment building to each case's residence and asking for volunteers.

1 Discuss the benefits and limitations of using a case-control design in this situation.

2 Interpret the investigators' main finding of an odds ratio of 4.50 (95% confidence interval: 1.20, 21.70) for exposure to live poultry in the market the week before illness, and consider the implications.

Conclusion

In this chapter you have reviewed the key features, advantages and disadvantages of case-control studies. This design takes the opposite approach to cohort studies, by determining outcome before exposure status, and therefore has a greater likelihood of bias. The population is not sampled randomly, so case-control studies cannot be used to estimate the incidence or prevalence of outcome or frequency of exposure. Case-control studies are generally cheaper and shorter than cohort studies, as they do not require any follow-up of participants. This design is especially useful for studying rare outcomes, or those with long latency periods.

References

Khoury MJ and Beaty TH (1994) Applications of the case-control method in genetic epidemiology. *Epidemiologic Reviews* 16: 134–50.

Moss AR, Osmond D, Bacchetti P, et al. (1987) Risk factors for AIDS and HIV seropositivity in homosexual men. *American Journal of Epidemiology* 125: 1035–47.

Mounts AW, Kwong H, Izurieta HS, et al. (1999) Case-control study of risk factors for avian influenza A (H5N1) disease, Hong Kong, 1997. *Journal of Infectious Diseases* 180: 505–8.

Rosenberg L, Metzger LS and Palmer JR (1993) Alcohol consumption and risk of breast cancer: a review of the epidemiologic evidence. *Epidemiologic Reviews* 15: 133–44.

Feedback on activities

Activity 9.1

1 A case-control design is superior in this example for several reasons. First, breast cancer is known to be associated with several risk factors and the case-control design

allows investigation of multiple exposures. Second, breast cancer has a long latent period and is relatively uncommon, so a cohort design would need more resources and time to follow up sufficient participants. Third, an ecological study would not be able to establish a causal link, though it could be used initially to generate the research question by indicating a possible link between breast cancer and alcohol.

Activity 9.2

1 (a) Women were interviewed within 6 months of diagnosis, so that only incident cases of breast cancer were included in the study. Inclusion of prevalent cases may lead to bias if as prevalent cases may have changed their behaviour and therefore their exposure to risk factors as a result of their disease. Restricting the study to incident cases also ensures that severe cases are not under-represented.

   (b) Although selection of population-based cases may result in a study that is less prone to bias, the logistics and costs involved may make it easier to identify cases in a hospital setting, particularly cases of a rare disease such as cancer. There is then the consideration of whether those with the disease under investigation are likely to be admitted to hospital. Women with breast cancer are almost certain to be referred or admitted to hospital once diagnosed, so selection of hospital-based cases is appropriate in this study.

2 In designing a questionnaire, you would consider what information is needed, and how you would ask questions to reduce potential measurement and recall bias. For example, it is well known that people tend to under-report their alcohol consumption.
   You might collect the following information related to alcohol consumption:
   • Whether the participant is a current, past, or non-drinker.
   • What type of alcohol they consume (e.g. beer, wine, spirits).
   • How much alcohol they consume (e.g. number of drinks per day).
   • How often they drink (e.g. number of days per week).
   • The age at which they started drinking (and age at which they stopped drinking, if they stopped).

   Other questions you would ask would elicit basic demographic information about the participants (e.g. date of birth, education, occupation). You would ask about potential confounders such as smoking and known risk factors for breast cancer (e.g. age at menarche, age at menopause, number of pregnancies, age at first birth).

3 In general, investigators find it convenient to select controls from the same setting in which they selected the cases. However, it is important that the study is not then biased by selecting controls that are more similar to cases in terms of exposure than they would have been if selected from the general population.
   Some hospital-based studies use two control groups, one from a hospital setting and the other from the population. If the selection of controls from within the hospital setting has not led to any bias, the results should not differ between the two control groups. However, if the results differ between the control groups, interpretation may be a problem.
   Any exclusion criteria that apply to cases should also apply to controls (e.g. women aged over 74 years, women with previous breast cancer). You may also consider excluding patients who are admitted to hospital with alcohol-related diseases, and diseases related to known risk factors for breast cancer (e.g. gynaecological diseases). Many case-control studies of a specific cancer also exclude controls with any sort of

cancer. In hospital-based studies, it is important to include controls with a range of different diseases so that no one disease is unduly represented.

4 The investigators could have matched on age. They could also have matched on a known risk factor for breast cancer such as parity (the number of times a woman has given birth). However, this would be more complicated and it is important not to overmatch (i.e. match on alcohol status by mistake).

5 The 30 women with breast cancer who were not included in the study may have differed from other cases in some way. This would lead to *selection bias* as the cases might not be representative of all women with breast cancer, especially if those not participating differed in relation to their alcohol consumption.

The investigators' knowledge of the hypothesis might have led to *observer bias*. The investigators may have asked more probing questions about alcohol use if the participant was a case.

The six interviewers may also have varied in the way they conducted the interview, or the way they recorded information, leading to *information bias*.

Biases could have been minimized by:
- blinding the interviewers to the study hypothesis;
- blinding the interviewers to the identity of the cases and controls;
- using a small number of interviewers to reduce inter-observer variation;
- using a structured questionnaire to avoid subjectivity on the part of the interviewer;
- training the interviewers and supervising some interviews to ensure consistency.

Activity 9.3

1 The case-control design is ideal for an outbreak situation as rapid results are needed. There are unlikely to be many prevalent cases, so a cross-sectional study would be inappropriate. It is not possible to predict the frequency of the outcome, and when first identified the outcome is likely to be rare, making it impractical to implement a cohort study.

However, there may be *selection bias* due to difficulties in identifying appropriate controls, especially if the risk factors have not yet been identified. The choice of neighbourhood controls could lead to overmatching if the risk factor is an environmental exposure, and several types of controls should be used in this situation to avoid this bias. There may be *information bias*, as the outcome status is already known. In this situation, where media coverage of the death had occurred and the source of the virus had been identified as birds, cases may have remembered their recent contact with live poultry differently to controls, thus biasing results.

2 As this is a case-control study, the measure of association is the odds ratio of *exposure*. This means that cases were four times more likely than controls to have had contact with live poultry in the week before the illness. It does *not* tell us that those who had contact with live poultry were four times more likely to suffer from H5N1 disease. However, while it is a useful indicator of the factors that may be associated with an outcome, this study does not provide sufficient evidence of causality for reasons mentioned in the previous answer.

Given the potential implications of identifying live poultry markets as the cause of the outbreak (e.g. slaughter of all poultry, closure of poultry markets), further supportive evidence would be needed (e.g. isolation of H5N1 virus from poultry in the markets) before inferring causality.

10 Intervention studies

Overview

The analytical study designs described in Chapters 6–9 are all observational, i.e. investigators observe the natural development of the outcome without interfering. Intervention studies are epidemiological experiments during which the investigators aim to change the natural occurrence of an outcome by manipulating the exposure. Both cross-sectional and cohort methods may be used to measure the relative frequency between exposure and outcome and consequently the effect of the introduced intervention. The randomized controlled trial (RCT) is the ideal intervention study design as it reduces error due to bias and confounding. Given ethical constraints, other intervention study designs may be used when a RCT is not acceptable. Intervention studies may measure intervention *efficacy* under ideal conditions or *effectiveness* under routine conditions.

Learning objectives

When you have completed this chapter you should be able to:

- describe the use, strengths and limitations of intervention studies
- distinguish between the different types of intervention study design
- recognize the basic analytical approaches used
- discuss ethical issues related to the design and conduct of intervention studies.

What defines an intervention study?

An intervention study measures the association between an outcome and exposure to a specific **intervention**. Interventions may focus on *prevention* of exposure in those at risk of the outcome (e.g. insecticide-treated mosquito nets against malaria) or *treatment* to reduce mortality or severity in those who already have the outcome (e.g. interferon treatment of people with chronic Hepatitis B to reduce progression to liver cancer). An intervention may remove or reduce an assumed risk factor (e.g. health education to reduce smoking), or it may introduce or increase an assumed protective factor (e.g. vaccination against poliovirus).

Either cohort or cross-sectional methods may be used to measure the relative frequency of the outcome in those exposed and unexposed to the intervention under study. However, unlike the observational study designs described previously, intervention studies are *experimental* because the investigators are able to *intervene*. In this design, the investigators define which study subjects are 'exposed' and which are 'unexposed'. For ethical reasons experimental studies are restricted to evaluating exposures that reduce the frequency of a negative outcome.

Advantages and disadvantages

The intervention study design is ideal for inferring causality (see Chapter 4) for the following reasons:

1 The exposure is defined prior to development of the outcome, so the temporal sequence is established, satisfying the *temporality* consideration for causality.
2 If the intervention is the removal or reduction of an exposure of interest that results in a reduction in the frequency of an outcome, it satisfies the *reversibility* consideration for causality.
3 Investigators are able to *randomize* study subjects to be exposed and unexposed to the intervention. If the number of subjects is large enough to reduce the effects of *chance*, this ensures that all known and unknown *confounders* are equally distributed between comparison groups (i.e. comparison groups are identical in all ways except for the intervention and there is no *selection bias*).
4 Investigators may be able to conceal the **allocation** of the intervention from study subjects and from those measuring the outcome, reducing *information bias*.

Intervention studies are not appropriate for very rare outcomes, as they generally use cohort methods that would require a long follow-up time. However, if the outcome is chronic (e.g. Hepatitis C infection) it may be possible to measure the intervention effect using cross-sectional surveys with very large sample sizes.

Intervention studies are often long and expensive to carry out. They may require a large study team and lengthy follow-up time to identify sufficient subjects with the outcome. There may also be additional costs of the intervention itself, as well as costs related to concealing the allocation and monitoring the safety of the intervention.

If an intervention is already in routine use, it may not be feasible to withdraw it from participants in the control group without providing an alternative, even if the safety or efficacy of the intervention is unknown or in doubt. For example, there is no evidence that prenatal ultrasound screening improves birth outcome and concerns have been raised about its potential long-term effects. However, routine ultrasound scans are an accepted part of obstetric care in developed countries and it would be difficult to recruit sufficient subjects to a randomized trial where routine ultrasound was withheld from the comparison group.

Ethical objections may be raised about withholding an intervention from the comparison group if the intervention has already been shown to be safe and effective in a previous study. However, it is not unusual for an initial study to show evidence of an effect, while subsequent studies in different settings give conflicting results. Ethical responsibility must be balanced against the need for sufficient and consistent epidemiological evidence, and a systematic review of existing evidence should be undertaken before developing any intervention study proposal.

Study design

Ethical approval

It is necessary to obtain 'ethical approval' (i.e. permission) from national and institutional ethical bodies prior to conducting any epidemiological investigation, but this is even more relevant to intervention studies as investigators determine which intervention the participants receive. The World Health Organization and other national and international bodies have developed guidelines for intervention studies based on the *Declaration of Helsinki*. However, whether a study is judged to be ethical can vary greatly between countries and over time, as scientific knowledge and cultural norms develop.

Intervention studies need to address questions of sufficient public health importance to justify their use. Ethical considerations will often drive the choice of specific study design (see below) as most designs involve the 'denial' of a *potentially* efficacious intervention to subjects allocated to the control arm during the study period. However, the general population will eventually benefit if the study provides sufficient evidence of a protective intervention effect, and those who participated in the trial should be the first to benefit from such an intervention once the trial is over.

Efficacy and effectiveness

There are two stages in evaluating an intervention that can be addressed using the intervention study design. *Efficacy* studies aim to measure the effect of the intervention under 'experimental' conditions, where maximum effort is put into intervention delivery. For example, participants in an infant vaccine trial may be reminded to attend for vaccination or even visited at home if they do not attend the vaccination clinic.

Once an intervention has been proven to be efficacious, it may be appropriate to undertake an *effectiveness* study to measure the effect of the intervention under routine conditions. This is especially important for interventions that rely on fragile delivery systems such as a weak health infrastructure, or where long-term patient compliance is required. The effectiveness of an intervention may be very different to its efficacy, and provides a better estimate of its likely impact when administered to the general population. In the infant vaccine example, effectiveness will depend on factors such as whether the vaccine is in stock and viable, whether infants attend for vaccination, their age when they attend, and the number of doses they receive. While the vaccine may have a 90% efficacy against the outcome, if only 50% of those at risk of the outcome actually receive sufficient doses of viable vaccine at the correct time, the effectiveness could be closer to 45% ($0.9 \times 0.5 = 0.45$).

Plausibility studies

Plausibility studies evaluate the *effectiveness* of interventions by comparison with a historical, geographical or opportunistic control group, but without randomization. They are appropriate in the following situations (Victora et al. 2004):

1. When an intervention is so complex that RCT results will be unacceptably artificial.
2. When an intervention is known to be efficacious or effective in small-scale studies, but its effectiveness on a large scale must be demonstrated.
3. When ethical concerns prevent the use of an RCT.

Historical controls

If it is not possible to have a contemporary comparison arm for ethical or logistical reasons, an intervention study may compare outcome frequency before and after the intervention is introduced. This design is most commonly used in evaluations of health services. However, the use of such 'historical' controls makes it difficult to distinguish the effect of the intervention from other changes that may have affected the outcome over the study period. If this design is used, it is necessary to carefully monitor other changes that may occur in the study population (e.g. migrations, introduction of other interventions, changes in climate variables), other outcomes that should not have been affected by the intervention, and the outcome of interest in the general population to which the intervention has not been applied.

Geographical controls

The use of communities or individuals as contemporary control from outside the trial area may adjust for the effects of temporal changes during the course of the evaluation. However, there are likely to be inherent differences between the control and intervention communities that need to be considered when interpreting the results.

A variant of this, which enables some randomization, is called the *stepped-wedge design*. It is not frequently used, because of the complexity of the design and logistics. The interventions may be phased in to a population over time, usually in line with practical delays in introducing a new intervention (e.g. training of health staff, community health education). In the first such trial, Hepatitis B vaccine was gradually introduced into The Gambia by adding a new immunization team responsible for a different part of the country every three months (The Gambia Hepatitis Study Group 1987). The order in which the

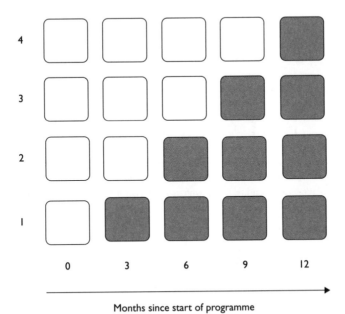

Figure 10.1 Schematic of stepped-wedge intervention trial design. Shaded squares represent clusters receiving the intervention. Unshaded squares represent clusters that have not yet received the intervention (controls). Over the course of the trial the total number of intervention and control clusters are equal, but the distribution varies with time

Source: Drawn by Ilona Carneiro, modified from The Gambia Hepatitis Study Group (1987) and Brown and Lilford (2006).

intervention was introduced was randomly allocated, and those areas that had not yet received the intervention acted as the control arm of the study (see Figure 10.1).

As the intervention and control arms are not equally distributed over time, any change in other risk factors for the outcome over the course of the study may confound the findings. This can be reduced by having large numbers of clusters and small interval periods for introduction of the intervention to each additional cluster.

Opportunistic controls

This involves the use of individuals or communities that should have received the intervention but did not because the programme was unable to reach them. If the controls have varying degrees of exposure to the intervention, it may be possible to measure a dose–response effect.

Randomized-controlled trials

While effectiveness studies may be subject to ethical and practical design limitations, an efficacy study is ideally conducted as a randomized-controlled trial (RCT). Trials in which the intervention is not randomly allocated are likely to suffer from selection bias and confounding, but may be used to provide preliminary evidence prior to a more rigorous study. RCTs are defined by: (a) the existence of a contemporary comparison group of study subjects who do not receive the intervention, known as the 'control' arm; and (b) the *random* allocation of study subjects to the intervention and control arms.

You may see the terms 'phase 2' or 'phase 3' applied to RCTs, especially where a clinical outcome is being measured. For example, a phase 3 RCT to evaluate the efficacy of insecticide-treated mosquito nets against malaria incidence. This classification comes from clinical trials of new medical interventions (e.g. drugs, vaccines, diagnostics, surgical procedures), which are conducted in several consecutive phases. Phase 1 trials apply the intervention to small numbers of healthy volunteers to assess issues such as safety and tolerability. Phase 2 trials evaluate efficacy and safety in larger groups of about 100–300 people, and may use the RCT design. Phase 3 clinical trials aim to provide definitive evidence of efficacy in individuals at risk of the outcome and usually use the RCT design. Phase 4 trials monitor the routine use of an intervention without a comparison group, mainly to collect data on safety (pharmacovigilance), and are akin to effectiveness studies and monitoring of routine health programmes (see Chapter 12).

Cluster-randomized trials

In **cluster-randomized** RCTs, groups of individuals known as 'clusters' are randomly allocated to the intervention and control arms, and all individuals within the same cluster receive the same intervention or control. This design may be used if the intervention acts at the cluster level (e.g. an intervention that reduces air pollution would need to be introduced at the community level since it would be impossible to introduce pollution controls at an individual level). Cluster randomization may be appropriate when there is a risk of *contamination* between the intervention and control groups, such that controls may be exposed to the intervention or vice versa. For example, in a trial of health education leaflets to promote healthy diet in school children, investigators would randomize at the school level. If they had randomized at the individual level, children within a particular school might show the leaflets to friends in the control group. Cluster-randomized trials require larger sample sizes as individuals within a cluster will share several characteristics and cannot be treated as independent observations, leading to reduced statistical power. Therefore, special methods are required to estimate sample sizes for cluster-randomized trials and to analyse the results (for more information see Hayes and Moulton 2009).

Factorial design

In a **factorial trial**, two or more interventions are compared individually and in combination against a control comparison group. This has the advantage of enabling us to assess interactions between interventions, and may save time and money by evaluating several intervention combinations simultaneously. For example we might want to compare the relative and additive efficacy of an insecticide-treated net (ITN) and intermittent preventive treatment for malaria in infants (ITPi) with sulphadoxine-pyrimethamine (SP) (see Figure 10.2). A factorial design would result in a four-arm trial: (i) infants in group 1 would receive an untreated mosquito net and an IPTi placebo-drug and would be the reference group; (ii) infants in group 2 would receive an untreated mosquito net and IPTi with SP, (iii) infants in group 3 would receive an ITN and an IPTi placebo-drug, and (iv) infants in group 4 would receive both an ITN and IPTi with SP.

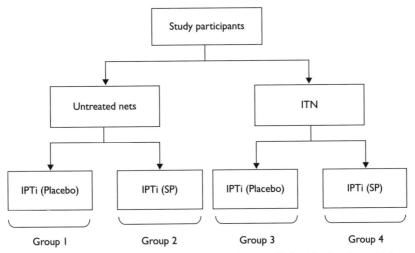

Figure 10.2 Flow-chart of a factorial design randomized controlled trial of an insecticide treated net (ITN) and/or intermittent preventive treatment in infants (IPTi) with sulphadoxine pyrimethamine (SP) or a placebo

Source: Ilona Carneiro, modified from LSHTM lecture notes.

Crossover design

In a **crossover** design RCT, each trial subject (e.g. individual, village) acts as its own control by receiving either the intervention or control at different points in the study, with a **washout period** (i.e. the time needed for the intervention to stop having an effect) to avoid contamination between the study periods. The order in which the subject receives the intervention or control (e.g. intervention then placebo, or placebo then intervention) is determined by random allocation. This design is only suitable when the intervention does not have long-term effects. However, it enables us to control for all confounders and effect modifiers.

The following specific study design issues refer to RCTs.

Sampling

As with all epidemiological studies, study participants should be representative of the population to which the intervention will ultimately be applied. Eligible subjects are identified using clearly defined inclusion and exclusion criteria and informed consent must be obtained (see Chapter 5).

There may be some selection bias at enrolment, especially if there is a risk of serious side-effects or a chance of not receiving active treatment for a medical condition. For example, an individual with asymptomatic chronic Hepatitis B infection might be less willing to join a trial of treatment to suppress viral replication than might an individual with abnormal liver function. Equally, individuals with advanced cancer that have already tried existing treatments may be more willing to try a new experimental treatment. Such selection may affect the estimate of efficacy if the intervention acts differently at different stages of disease, and it may not be appropriate to generalize the result to the wider target population.

Selection bias may also be introduced during the course of the study If there is a difference in the follow-up between the intervention arms. For example, participants may be more likely to withdraw from a study if there are side effects or if they feel the intervention is not working. There may also be differences in compliance due to clinical deterioration or because a participant forgets to administer a placebo because they do not notice any benefit (e.g. a placebo mosquito repellent). Participants who are lost to follow-up or do not comply may be different from those who complete the study, and baseline data on important risk factors should be compared to assess the potential for selection bias. The proportions of subjects lost to follow-up and those not included in the final analysis must also be compared between the different intervention arms to identify any selection bias.

Choice of control

Participants receiving the intervention of interest are compared to those not receiving the intervention of interest, called the **control** arm. Comparison will vary according to the intervention being evaluated, and subjects in the control arm may receive nothing, a **placebo** intervention, or an existing intervention. Typically, we want to know the effect of an intervention compared with current practice. If no intervention is currently in use, the control arm may receive no intervention, but should otherwise have identical access to all the treatment and preventive services as those in the intervention arm.

Investigators may use a placebo, a simulated intervention with no active properties, as a negative control in intervention studies, because the act of receiving an intervention may itself affect a subject's perceived or actual outcome. An individual who thinks they are receiving a treatment may actually experience a reduction in symptoms. This positive outcome without any active intervention is known as the *placebo effect*. A study subject may also experience more negative effects (i.e. increased symptoms or side-effects) after receiving a placebo, which is known as the *nocebo effect*.

These responses have been shown to have a neurobiological basis in brain imaging studies, but they are not yet fully understood. For some outcomes (e.g. Parkinson's disease, irritable bowel syndrome), self-healing processes were identified as playing a role after a placebo intervention was shown to have an effect. In epidemiology, the use of a placebo enables us to adjust for the 'background' effects of participating in the trial, such as participant expectation, interaction with study investigators and tests for monitoring and measuring the outcome.

Where an intervention already exists, it would be unethical to withdraw the existing intervention in exchange for a placebo. The control arm participants must receive the best current drug or practice available to them, although this may not always be the best available worldwide. For example, studies in country X find drug A to be a better treatment for tuberculosis than the existing drug B, and drug A is implemented as the new first-line therapy in countries X and Y. However, no studies have yet been undertaken in country Z where drug B is still the first-line therapy. Investigators may successfully argue for a RCT of drug A compared with drug B in country Z, as control participants will be receiving the best *available* current practice. However, it would no longer be possible to carry out the same trial in country Y, even if there were no prior local evidence, because drug A is already the best treatment currently available to study participants.

Allocation

Allocation of participants is usually done randomly so that any study participant has an equal chance of being allocated to the intervention or control arms, therefore avoiding *selection bias* (see Chapter 4). If the sample size is sufficiently large, this randomization ensures that any known or unknown *confounding* factors are equally distributed between study arms and will not interfere with an estimate of intervention effect.

Random allocation can be undertaken using similar methods to those described for random sampling in Chapter 5:

- *Simple randomization* uses random number tables or a computer-generated random number list. However, this could result in different numbers of subjects in each study arm.
- *Systematic randomization* allocates participants to each group alternately (e.g. on specific days), but this may be subject to selection bias. For example, there may be systematic differences in the severity of patients presenting to a clinic on a Monday (after the weekend) and those presenting on a Tuesday.
- *Blocked randomization* restricts the allocation list to ensure equal numbers in all study arms. For example, a trial comparing interventions A and B may use blocks of four to generate six possible randomization sequences with equal allocation: AABB, ABAB, BABA, ABBA, BAAB, BBAA. Blocks can then be chosen at random to define the allocation sequence but the investigator should not know the block size, as they might be able to predict the allocation for the last few participants in each block. Block size must be a multiple of the number of intervention arms, but large blocks should be avoided.
- *Stratified randomization* divides participants into subgroups or strata based on key risk factors (e.g. age, gender), and equal numbers of subjects from each stratum are randomly allocated to each study arm. This ensures that suspected confounders or effect modifiers of the association between intervention and outcome are equally

distributed between comparison groups. For example, malaria incidence varies considerably between communities due to socio-economic and geographic differences. In a RCT of an infant malaria vaccine, infants should be stratified according to their village of residence and allocation of the intervention based on block-randomization within village. This allows the investigators to control for village-level differences in malaria risk and other factors, which could otherwise vary by chance between the study arms.

• *Matched-pair randomization* is a form of stratified random allocation that matches individuals or communities into pairs with similar baseline risks of the outcome.

In small trials when several variables need to be balanced between study arms, stratified randomization is not sufficient to ensure comparability. Differences between study arms may still occur by chance, making it difficult to interpret results, even after adjusting for these differences in the analysis. In this situation, rather than randomly allocating subjects we purposefully allocate subjects based on a pre-specified list of criteria. This is known as **minimization**, as the intention is to minimize differences between study arms. As each subject is enrolled, their allocation depends on the characteristics of those subjects already enrolled (for further details see Altman and Bland 2005).

For all the methods described above there is a chance of conscious or unconscious *selection bias* if a study investigator undertakes the allocation. For example, they may tend to allocate more seriously affected patients to the intervention and less seriously affected patients to the control arm. To avoid such bias, the allocation sequence should be concealed from those enrolling study subjects.

Allocation concealment may use sealed envelopes determining the allocation, which are only opened after an eligible subject has consented to enter the trial. For multi-centre trials, there may be a centralized system where subject details are entered into the trial computer, which then randomly allocates the subject to one of the treatment groups. Another method is for allocation to be done by the manufacturer of the intervention (e.g. drug, vaccine, mosquito net), with the intervention and control packaged identically with serial numbers whose coding is known only to the manufacturer. Allocation concealment is not the same as blinding (see below). It is possible to conceal the allocation sequence prior to allocation in all RCTs, even though it may not then be possible to conceal it from subjects or observers after the allocation has been made.

Blinding

An 'open-label' trial is one in which participants and investigators are aware of which intervention is allocated to which study subjects. However, if a participant knows whether they are receiving a new intervention, existing intervention or placebo, it may affect their behaviour during the trial or their response to questions that aim to determine outcome. For example, a mother who knows her child was vaccinated against measles may be less likely to seek treatment for a fever than one whose child was not. If one of the study outcomes is clinic attendance with fever, this could result in **ascertainment bias** between the study arms. This is of greater concern if the outcome may be subjective, such as reported improvement in symptoms of multiple sclerosis.

Observer bias can also occur if the person assessing the outcome is aware of the allocation. For example, a microscopist reading blood slides to detect malaria parasites may be less thorough if they read the slides while sitting in a village with insecticide-treated curtains in every doorway than in one without curtains. For most outcomes it is usually possible to 'blind' the observer, i.e. to conceal the intervention allocation from the person diagnosing the outcome.

Use of a placebo intervention can help to conceal the allocation. While a placebo is easier to develop for drugs and vaccines it is not impossible to develop placebos for non-chemical interventions such as counselling or acupuncture. For example, 'sham' surgery maintains the illusion of an operation by using real anaesthesia, surgical incision and pre- and postoperative care, but leaving-out the actual intervention of interest. While this raises many ethical concerns, the increasing use of minimally invasive procedures (e.g. keyhole surgery) reduces negative effects for the participants while enabling a more rigorous testing of such interventions.

If either participant or observer is blinded, the study is *single-blind*, whereas if both are blinded, the study is *double-blind*. The 'gold standard' for RCTs is the *double-blind, randomized placebo-controlled trial*.

Data collection

Data collection methods in an intervention trial will be the same as for cohort or cross-sectional studies, depending on the design used. However, if the study has been blinded to those observing the outcome, it is important that intervention allocation is also blinded to those entering and analysing the data, to prevent any intentional or unintentional bias from being introduced.

Analysis

It is good practice for a statistician independent of the study team to hold the codes to the intervention allocation. Codes should not be revealed to study investigators until after data have been entered and cleaned. In large clinical trials, the data are 'frozen', i.e. a copy of the data prior to 'breaking-the-code' is sent to an independent statistician for safekeeping, to ensure that data are not changed after the allocation is revealed.

A detailed analytical plan should be developed prior to breaking the allocation codes. This will state the primary outcome of interest, any secondary outcomes of interest, the methods of analysis to be used (e.g. logistic regression models) and any variables to be adjusted for in the analysis. This prevents investigators from searching through the data and only presenting positive results.

Interim analysis

In intervention studies with a long follow-up period, where there may be a possibility of severe adverse events, it is usual to have an independent trial safety monitoring board. This board is responsible for periodically reviewing all reports of severe adverse events. If there is a concern about greater than expected numbers of adverse events in one study arm, the board will analyse the data and if necessary the trial will be stopped. It is also common for the monitoring board to undertake an independent **interim analysis** of the data halfway through a long study. If there is sufficient epidemiological evidence that the intervention is working, or that the trial will have insufficient power to detect an effect, the trial may also be interrupted.

Intention-to-treat vs. per-protocol

The primary analysis of an intervention study should be by **intention-to-treat** (ITT). This means that the outcome is compared between study participants according to the groups to which they were allocated at the start of the study, even if they changed groups, withdrew from the study or were lost to follow-up. ITT maintains the original allocation to ensure comparability between intervention arms, and avoids potential selection biases that can arise from different levels of participation during the study. For example, assume that the side-effects of cancer treatment X caused more advanced-stage patients to deteriorate more rapidly and be withdrawn from the study prior to completing treatment. Excluding them from the analysis might result in more severe cases in the comparison arm at the end of the study, mistakenly implying that treatment X was more effective than the control.

The ITT estimate of intervention effect will be closer to what may result in the 'real world', where individuals may not all receive the intervention at the prescribed time points or may not use the interventions as intended. However, we might also want to know what the 'true potential' of the intervention might be in an ideal world (e.g. if we were able to improve delivery or compliance). For this reason, a secondary analysis may be carried out **per-protocol**. In per-protocol analysis, only those study participants who receive the intervention according to the pre-defined protocol are included in the analysis. For example, a vaccine trial may specify vaccination of infants between 6–10 weeks, 10–14 weeks and 14–18 weeks of age. Including infants in the analysis who missed doses or who received doses very late will lead to *non-differential misclassification bias* and may underestimate the potential of the vaccine.

Intervention efficacy

Once the intervention allocation has been revealed, the baseline data (e.g. age, sex, ethnic group, disease grade) are compared between intervention arms to show how successful the allocation process was in producing comparable participants. Differences in baseline characteristics may be due to chance or to biases in the allocation method. If differences are considered to be due to chance, they may be adjusted for by including these factors in a multivariable regression model, for example. If the differences may be due to biased allocation, then it will not be possible to interpret whether any differences are due to the intervention or to selection bias.

As intervention studies generally use cohort methods, the measures of association are risk and rate ratios (see Chapter 3). Some intervention studies may also measure prevalence as a secondary outcome using cross-sectional surveys, and the odds ratio may be calculated as an estimate of the prevalence ratio (see Chapter 7).

The *efficacy* of an intervention is calculated as the proportion of cases that can be prevented by the intervention. This is also known as the *protective efficacy* or *preventable fraction* and is the inverse of the attributable fraction (see Chapter 3). *Intervention efficacy* is calculated as:

Intervention efficacy = 1 − Relative risk

Interpretation

As with all epidemiological studies, the results need to be interpreted with caution, considering the roles of chance, bias and confounding. However, if the trial has been conducted correctly with effective allocation and blinding procedures, and it has sufficient statistical power, these alternative explanations are unlikely to unduly influence the estimated measure of intervention effect. Even if we can infer a causal relationship between exposure to the intervention and frequency of outcome, additional factors such as adverse effects, delivery, cost and acceptability of the intervention all need to be evaluated before an intervention is considered for implementation.

Activity 10.1

In The Gambia, infants aged 6–51 weeks who presented to a government vaccination post were screened for eligibility and written parental consent obtained for inclusion in an intervention study. Some 17,437 children were randomly allocated to receive three doses of either pneumococcal vaccine or a placebo with intervals of at least 25 days between doses (Cutts et al. 2005). They were subsequently monitored for pneumonia over 24 months through attendance at the local health facilities and hospital. An independent contractor had labelled vaccine and placebo vials with code numbers using a blocked design and unique study identity numbers. These numbers were subsequently used on health cards, and after the third vaccination had been received, there was no record of the randomization code on the health card.

1 What type of study is this? Be as specific as you can.
2 The results presented included only those children who received the first dose when aged 40–364 days with at least 25 days' interval between doses. What type of analysis is this and which children might have been excluded from the analysis?
3 The incidence rate for first episode of radiological pneumonia was 26.0 per 1,000 child years in infants who received the vaccine and 40.9 in infants who received the placebo. Calculate and name an appropriate measure of effect, showing details of your calculations, and interpret your result.
4 The investigators state: 'Efficacy did not vary by age ...'. Given the information presented in Table 10.1, do you agree with their interpretation? Give reasons for your answer.

Table 10.1 Vaccine efficacy against first episode of invasive pneumococcal disease

Age (months)	% Vaccine efficacy (95% CI)
3–11	93 (54, 100)
12–23	75 (32, 93)
24–29	26 (–339, 89)

Source: Cutts et al. (2005).

Activity 10.2

A (fictitious) study was carried out on the maternity ward of ten hospitals to test the effect of oral versus intramuscular vitamin K to reduce clinical bleeding in newborns. After obtaining informed parental consent, children born on odd-numbered days received doses of 2.0 mg oral vitamin K on days 1 and 3 after birth. Children born on

even-numbered days constituted the control group and received 1.0 mg of intramuscular vitamin K the day after birth according to existing practice. All infants were followed
up to assess spontaneous bleeding on days 1–7 after birth.

1 What type of study is this? Be as specific as you can.
2 Discuss the potential limitations of this design and ways in which it might be
  improved.

Activity 10.3

A multi-centre double-blind randomized placebo-controlled trial in 274 hospitals
across 40 countries was undertaken to assess whether early administration of tranexamic acid to 20,211 adult trauma patients with haemorrhage could reduce the risk
of death in hospital within 4 weeks of injury. Data were analysed by time from injury to
treatment, and found that the relative risk of death due to bleeding was 0.68 (95%
confidence interval (CI): 0.57, 0.82) if treatment occurred within 1 hour, 0.79 (95% CI:
0.64, 0.97) if treatment occurred within 1–3 hours, and 1.44 (95% CI: 1.12, 1.84) if
treatment occurred three or more hours after trauma (Roberts et al. 2011).

1 Interpret these results referring to the study design used, and give your recommendations for the use of tranexamic acid based on these data.
2 In some cases, the injury was not witnessed and the time interval between injury and
  treatment was estimated. How might this have affected the results?

Activity 10.4

Intermittent preventive treatment for malaria in infants (IPTi) is a single curative dose
of an anti-malarial drug given to infants at routine vaccination clinic contacts regardless
of symptoms or malaria infection. A study randomly selected 12 out of 24 sub-districts
in rural Tanzania to introduce IPTi through the existing health infrastructure (Armstrong
Schellenberg et al. 2010).

A representative sample of 600 infants surveyed a year later using rapid diagnostic
tests (dipsticks) found 31% infected with malaria in the intervention sub-districts and
38% in the comparison sub-districts ($P = 0.06$). A comparison of only those infants who
had received IPTi and/or routine vaccination 2–6 weeks prior to the survey found 22%
malaria infection in the intervention sub-districts compared with 41% in the comparison sub-districts ($P = 0.01$).

1 What type of study design is this? Be as specific as you can.
2 Identify the two approaches to analysis that were undertaken and describe their
  results. What does a comparison of these results imply about implementation of IPTi?

Conclusion

In this chapter you have reviewed the key features, advantages and disadvantages of
intervention studies. The experimental nature of this type of study raises many ethical
concerns that subsequently drive the specific choice of study design. Intervention

studies are generally more complex and costly than other study designs. However, intervention studies are less likely to suffer from bias and confounding, and are usually the design of choice for producing relevant public health evidence.

References

Altman DG and Bland JM (2005) Treatment allocation by minimisation. *British Medical Journal* 330: 843.

Armstrong Schellenberg JR, Shirima K, Maokola W, et al. (2010) Community effectiveness of intermittent preventive treatment for infants (IPTi) in rural southern Tanzania. *American Journal of Tropical Medicine and Hygiene* 82: 772–81.

Brown CA and Lilford RJ (2006) The stepped wedge trial design: a systematic review. *BMC Medical Research Methodology* 6: 54.

Cutts FT, Zaman SM, Enwere G, et al. (2005) Efficacy of nine-valent pneumococcal conjugate vaccine against pneumonia and invasive pneumococcal disease in The Gambia: randomised, double-blind, placebo-controlled trial. *Lancet* 365: 1139–46.

Hayes RJ and Moulton LH (2009) *Cluster Randomised Trials*. Boca Raton, FL: Chapman and Hall/CRC Press.

Roberts I, Shakur H, Afolabi A, et al. (2011) The importance of early treatment with tranexamic acid in bleeding trauma patients: an exploratory analysis of the CRASH-2 randomised controlled trial. *Lancet* 377: 1096–101, 1101–12.

The Gambia Hepatitis Study Group (1987) The Gambia Hepatitis Intervention Study. *Cancer Research* 47: 5782–7.

Victora CG, Habicht JP and Bryce J (2004) Evidence-based public health: moving beyond randomized trials. *American Journal of Public Health* 94: 400–5.

Feedback for activities

Activity 10.1

1 This is a double-blind, randomized placebo-controlled trial of pneumococcal vaccine in infants in The Gambia. 'Double-blind' because allocation codes and unique identifiers were used so that neither the parents of the infants nor the health personnel assessing the outcomes were aware of the allocation. 'Randomized' because there was an equal chance of any infant being in either study arm. 'Placebo-controlled' because the infants in the comparison group received an identical vaccine that had no active properties against any outcome.

2 This is a per-protocol analysis as it includes only those who received the intervention as it was originally intended. This analysis would exclude children who were less than 6 weeks or greater than 52 weeks (1 year) old when they received the first dose, those who had less than 25 days between either the first and second or second and third doses, those who did not receive all three doses, and those who may have received the vaccine instead of the placebo or the placebo instead of the vaccine at any of the three doses. Those who withdrew or died during the study after receiving all doses would still be able to contribute person-time at risk for the period that they were in the study, and would not be excluded from a per-protocol analysis.

3 As this is an intervention study, the appropriate measure of effect would be the vaccine efficacy, which is calculated as 1 − relative risk. As the reported frequency of the outcome is an incidence rate, the appropriate measure of relative risk is the incidence rate ratio (IRR):

$$\text{IRR} = \frac{\text{Incidence rate in infants receiving vaccine}}{\text{Incidence rate in infants receiving placebo}} = \frac{26.0}{40.9} = 0.6357$$

The vaccine efficacy is calculated as $1 - 0.6357 = 0.3643$ or 36%. A vaccine efficacy of 36% means that 36% of episodes of radiological pneumonia in young children in The Gambia can be prevented by vaccination with three doses of the pneumococcal vaccine.

4 You may have stated that you disagree with the authors' interpretation because the estimates of vaccine efficacy are clearly different for each age group. The efficacy appears to decrease substantially with age, and vaccine efficacy is no longer significant in 24–29-month-old children as the 95% confidence interval includes zero. However, this is an incomplete interpretation of the results.

The authors' statement is in fact correct. The 95% confidence intervals are relatively wide and overlap between all age groups. This tells us that the estimates of vaccine efficacy are not significantly different between the age groups using a 5% probability cut-off. The difference in the point estimates of vaccine efficacy are likely to be due to a reduced statistical power to detect an effect in older age groups where the sample size may have been too small or the underlying incidence of invasive pneumococcal disease may have been lower.

Activity 10.2

1 This is a multi-centre, open-label (non-blinded), systematically randomized-controlled trial. 'Multi-centre' because subjects were recruited and followed up in several study sites (hospitals). 'Open-label' because the parents of the infants and those administering the intervention will be aware of whether the infant receives an injection or an oral supplement. It is also likely a clinician recording the outcome would be aware of the child's date of birth and could therefore determine the allocation group. 'Systematically randomized' because the intervention allocation depends on the day a child was born and is not totally random, neither is it non-random, because there is usually no choice (either from the parents or the investigators) about the day a child is born unless it is a scheduled caesarean delivery. 'Controlled' because there is a comparison group that receives the existing intervention (not a placebo intervention).

2 You may have identified the following potential limitations:

(a) 'Open-label': The study is not blinded, so that parents of infants and those administering the intervention are aware of which intervention is received by a particular infant. Even the person recording bleeding events may be aware of the allocation as they will observe the child's date of birth on the medical charts. Knowledge of the intervention allocation may affect a parent's report of adverse events, or a clinician's diagnosis of outcome. It would not be justifiable to use a placebo injectable on a newborn, and even if a placebo oral supplement were used, it would not be ethical to withdraw the existing injectable intervention from the control arm participants. Therefore, the study outcomes would need to be very clearly defined (e.g. amount of bleeding) to reduce subjectivity and potential *information bias*.

(b) 'Systematic allocation': The allocation is systematic so that, even if a placebo had been used, investigators could determine the intervention allocation from the child's date of birth. However, children born on odd- or even-numbered days are unlikely to differ in any way and the two groups should still be sufficiently similar to control for any confounding factors. Given that the study is open-label, systematic allocation of the intervention is unlikely to result in any further bias.

(c) As this is an intervention in newborn children, there may be a high proportion of parents refusing to participate in the study. Alternatively, if injectable vitamin K is routinely given without the need for parental consent, parents may prefer to participate in the study to have a 50% chance of the less invasive oral intervention instead. If parents providing informed consent to participate in the trial differ from those who do not, this may affect our ability to extrapolate these results to the general population.

Activity 10.3

1 The protective efficacy of tranexamic acid given within one hour of injury is $1 - 0.68 = 0.32$, between 1–3 hours is $1 - 0.79 = 0.21$ and after three hours or more is $1 - 1.44 = -0.44$. This means treatment with tranexamic can reduce the risk of deaths due to bleeding by 32% if given within one hour of injury, by 21% if given within 1–3 hours of injury and will *increase* the risk of death by 44% if given more than three hours after injury.

   The 95% confidence intervals for all three relative risks do not include one, meaning that these estimates are significant at the 5% level. Given the size of the study, it is unlikely that these results could be due to chance. The trial was randomized, so it is unlikely that these results could be explained by confounding factors that varied between the study arms. As this was a double-blind trial, there is unlikely to be any information bias that would affect these estimates.

   Given the strength of evidence, the recommendation would be that tranexamic acid should be given as early as possible to bleeding trauma patients. However, tranexamic acid may be harmful for those admitted late after injury (Roberts et al. 2011).

2 If there were inaccuracies in estimating the time between injury and treatment, this would have led to misclassification of some individuals into the incorrect category of time to treatment. However, this should not have varied between study arms as the intervention allocation was randomized and blind. Any inaccuracies would therefore have led to *non-differential misclassification* of time-to-treatment, which may have diluted the association between intervention and outcome, underestimating the relative risks for each category.

Activity 10.4

1 This is an open-label, cluster-randomized, controlled effectiveness study of intermittent preventive treatment for malaria in infants. 'Open-label (non-blinded)' because there was no placebo intervention and both the communities involved and the study investigators determining the prevalence would have been aware of the intervention allocation (Note, if malaria infection had been determined by microscopy, it may have been possible to 'blind' the microscopist to the intervention allocation, however, the use of rapid diagnostic tests meant that infection status was determined *in situ* and investigators would have been aware of the sub-district allocation.) 'Cluster' because the units of randomization are sub-districts. 'Randomized' because the sub-districts were randomly selected to receive IPTi or not. 'Controlled' because there was a contemporary comparison arm of sub-districts that did not receive the intervention of interest. 'Effectiveness' because the intervention was delivered through the routine health system and not as part of a rigorous trial.

2 The first result of prevalence among infants in intervention compared with non-intervention sub-districts is an *intention-to-treat* analysis, where all infants were included according to whether the intervention was available in their sub-district,

and regardless of whether they had received it. The prevalence ratio of malaria infection for those receiving IPTi was $0.31 \div 0.38 = 0.815$ meaning that those in the IPTi communities had a 19% ($1 - 0.815 = 0.185$) lower likelihood of being infected than those in the control communities. A P-value of 0.06 means that, given the sample size and underlying prevalence, there is a 6% probability that this difference in prevalence might have been detected by chance if it was not real.

The second result was a *per-protocol* analysis, including only those infants who had actually received the intervention (or attended for routine vaccination in the control arm). The prevalence ratio was $0.22 \div 0.41 = 0.537$ meaning that those in the IPTi communities had a 46% ($1 - 0.537 = 0.463$) lower likelihood of being infected than those in the control communities. This result showed a statistically significant reduction ($P = 0.01$) in malaria prevalence in those infants who had recently received the intervention compared to those who had not.

The difference between the intention-to-treat and per-protocol results suggests that while the *efficacy* of IPTi was good in this setting, its *effectiveness* was not. These results suggest that, in this setting, the delivery of the intervention would need to be improved for it to have an important effect.

SECTION 3

Epidemiology in public health

Prevention strategies

Overview

In the previous chapters you learned how to measure epidemiological associations between an exposure and outcome, and to estimate the impact of a risk factor. In this chapter we consider how to apply such evidence to different approaches to preventive intervention. You will be introduced to the concepts of primary, secondary and tertiary prevention, and how the shape of the relationship between exposure and outcome influences whether to use a population or high-risk approach to targeting prevention. Screening is a key tool for prevention programmes and you will learn about the measures of sensitivity and specificity used to assess validity of a screening method and predictive values used to assess its utility at an individual level. We assess the main criteria necessary to evaluate whether a screening programme should be implemented.

Learning objectives

When you have completed this chapter you should be able to:

- define strategies in terms of primary, secondary and tertiary prevention
- recognize the importance of different dose–response relationships for prevention
- calculate measures of sensitivity, specificity and predictive values of a screening method
- explain the relationship between prevalence and predictive values
- list criteria for assessing the appropriateness of a screening programme
- distinguish between population and high-risk targeting, and identify the most appropriate prevention strategy for a given situation.

Prevention strategies

In previous chapters you learned about conducting rigorous epidemiological research studies, and how to evaluate epidemiological results. When there is satisfactory evidence that modification of an exposure can affect the frequency of an outcome, such data can be used to promote good health and prevent or reduce adverse outcomes. There are three main opportunities for preventive intervention relating to the natural development stages of an outcome (see Figure 11.1).

Primary prevention aims to stop an outcome developing, either by preventing or reducing exposure to a risk factor (e.g. vaccination against an infectious disease). When provided with information on risks, individuals can choose to modify behaviour, such as decreasing their weekly alcohol intake. At a population level, this may require societal changes in attitude or even legislation. For example, in Europe, health education

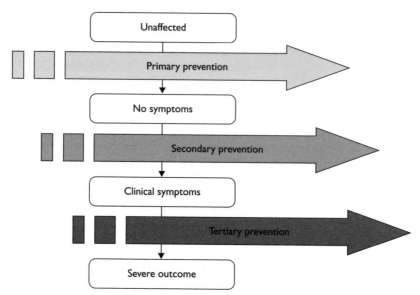

Figure 11.1 General outcome process illustrating the three levels at which intervention for prevention can act

Source: Ilona Carneiro.

campaigns were used to discourage the uptake and continued use of tobacco, then regulation of advertising and increased taxation of tobacco products was introduced, and finally laws prohibiting smoking in public places to reduce passive smoking (exposure to second-hand tobacco smoke).

Secondary prevention aims to interrupt progression from early to mid-stage of the outcome, mainly by early detection and prompt treatment. An individual may be unaware of having acquired an outcome because they have no symptoms or have not noticed the effects. Knowledge of the natural history of an outcome can help development of screening methods to detect the outcome early – this is a major component of secondary prevention. For example, childhood lead poisoning from house paint or industrial sites can cause seizures, coma and death. In the USA, blood lead screening identifies children at risk while they still have low blood lead levels.

Once the outcome is established and symptomatic, **tertiary prevention** aims to reduce complications or severity by offering appropriate treatments and interventions. For example, renal disease and glaucoma, both complications of uncontrolled diabetes, may be prevented in the diabetic patient if blood glucose levels are successfully regulated through the use of insulin and/or dietary restrictions.

For an outcome such as skin cancer, primary prevention might consist of health promotion campaigns to encourage people to reduce their exposure to the sun (e.g. using sun protection creams and protective clothing). Secondary prevention would focus on detecting and removing skin cancer lesions as soon as they occur to prevent development of invasive melanoma, sentinel lymph node biopsy to assess whether the cancer has spread, and regular check-ups to monitor recurrence. Tertiary prevention would include removal of any affected lymph nodes to prevent further cancer spread, and chemotherapy or radiotherapy to improve prognosis if the cancer has already spread.

Dose–response profiles

Prevention strategies may focus on those considered to be at highest risk of an outcome, or they may apply the intervention to the whole population. It does not make sense to target interventions at those who are not 'at risk'. In this chapter, the term 'population' refers to those generally at risk, as distinct from those at highest risk of an outcome.

To decide which approach is most appropriate we need to understand how the exposure relates to the outcome. Doctors typically classify people as being 'well' or 'unwell', as this helps decision-making about whether or not to admit a patient, prescribe a drug, or perform an operation. However, this approach provides little recognition of the disease process and how it manifests in populations. For many outcomes there is a range of poor health that may be related to a range of exposures to a risk factor. This is known as the 'dose–response' relationship, i.e. how the risk of outcome varies with changes in the measure of exposure (see Figure 11.2). For example, body mass index (or BMI, i.e. weight in kilogrammes divided by the square of height in metres) may result in poor health outcomes for those at very low levels or very high levels. Promoting an intervention to reduce BMI in the whole population could therefore negatively affect individuals with an already low BMI.

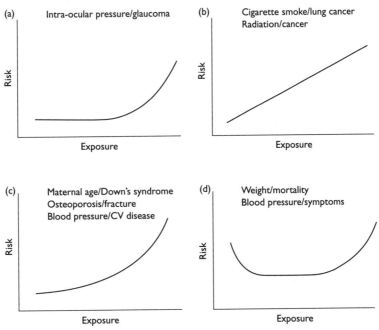

Figure 11.2 Schematic models of four different relationships between exposure to a risk factor and risk of outcome

Source: adapted from Rose (1992).

Alcohol and heart disease is another example. High alcohol intake may increase the risk of heart disease and other health problems (e.g. violence, road traffic accidents, etc.). However, there is some evidence to suggest that modest alcohol intake may have a protective effect on the risk of heart disease. It is therefore desirable to encourage people to reduce their alcohol intakes, but perhaps undesirable to encourage them to take no alcohol. In such cases, health promotion messages to the whole population need to be more sophisticated and complex, which may make it more difficult to appropriately inform people and encourage healthy behaviour.

The shape of the dose–response profile therefore has an important influence on our choice of prevention strategy. In Activity 11.1, you will look more closely at different dose–response profiles and consider their implications for prevention strategies.

Activity 11.1

1 Figure 11.2 provides four simplified 'dose–response' graphs. For each graph, briefly describe the relationship between exposure and outcome and the implications for the prevention strategy.

Screening

As you saw from Activity 11.1, it may be appropriate to target those at highest risk of an adverse outcome when the dose–response curve is not constant. Methods to identify individuals at greater risk of an outcome include physical examination, blood test, X-ray, and biopsy. **Screening** aims to identify small numbers of individuals at high risk of an outcome, whereas **diagnosis** is used to confirm outcome. The use of screening assumes that effective interventions are available to reduce risk, or to effectively treat an outcome that is detected sufficiently early. For example, screening individuals for high blood cholesterol levels aims to identify those at higher risk of coronary heart disease for targeted health promotion or cholesterol-lowering drug treatment. Screening may also be used for other purposes, including selection of people fit enough for a job, or containment of infection (e.g. screening new nurses or teachers for tuberculosis or food handlers for salmonella).

Screening can either include the whole population (*mass* screening) or selected groups who are expected to have a higher risk of exposure or outcome (*targeted* screening). A survey to measure the blood cholesterol of all adults in a population would be an example of mass screening. Targeted screening might only measure blood cholesterol in the relatives of people with familial hypercholesterolaemia (a high cholesterol genetic disorder).

Opportunistic screening may occur when a patient visits a healthcare provider and is offered screening unrelated to the reason for their visit. For example, a general medical practitioner may habitually take and record patients' blood pressure at the start of every consultation, or may offer all sexually active patients under 25 years of age a test for Chlamydia infection.

Systematic screening refers to an organized health programme (e.g. all women in the UK aged 25–64 are reminded to attend for a Papanicolaou cervical smear test every three years).

A screening method should ideally be inexpensive, easy to administer, and impose minimal discomfort on those to whom it is administered, given that a large proportion of those screened may not be at risk of adverse outcome. More importantly, the screening method (e.g. ultrasound scan, laboratory test, clinical definition) must correctly identify those at risk.

Sensitivity and specificity

The validity of a screening method is its ability to correctly distinguish between individuals with and without the condition of interest (i.e. risk factor, precursor, outcome). The validity of a screening method (or diagnostic test) is evaluated by calculating its **sensitivity** and **specificity**. An ideal screening method would have a high sensitivity and high specificity.

Table 11.1 Standard cross-tabulation (2 × 2 table) of true condition by screening/diagnostic result

		True condition		
		Present	Absent	Total
Screening Result	Positive	a	b	a + b
	Negative	c	d	c + d
	Total	a + c	b + d	a + b + c + d

Source: Ilona Carneiro.

In Table 11.1 we compare the distribution of screening method results in relation to the true condition of an individual:

- a represents the 'true positives' (i.e. the number who have the condition and have a positive result using the screening method);
- b represents the 'false positives' (i.e. the number of individuals who do not have the condition but have a positive result using the screening method);
- c represents the 'false negatives' (i.e. the number of individuals who have the condition but have a negative result using the screening method);
- d represents the 'true negatives' (i.e. the number of individuals who do not have the condition and have a negative result using the screening method).

The true condition of an individual may be determined either by a 'gold standard' diagnostic test (i.e. providing a definitive diagnosis), using the best existing alternative screening method, or by follow-up to assess final outcome. Where the screening method provides a continuous variable (e.g. blood glucose levels for diabetes), this must be categorized into a binomial variable using a defined cut-off based on previous evidence.

Sensitivity is the proportion of those who truly have the condition who are correctly identified ('true positives'). Referring to the notation in Table 11.1, sensitivity is calculated as:

$$\text{Sensitivity} = \frac{\textbf{Number of true positives}}{\textbf{Total number with the condition}} = \frac{a}{a + c}$$

Specificity is defined as the proportion of those who truly do not have the condition who are correctly identified ('true negatives'). Using the notation in Table 11.1, specificity is calculated as:

$$\text{Specificity} = \frac{\textbf{Number of true negatives}}{\textbf{Total number without the condition}} = \frac{d}{b + d}$$

The sensitivity and specificity values for a given method are usually not equal, and the relative importance of each depends on the outcome of interest. A low sensitivity means that the screening method results in many 'false negatives' (i.e. it would identify many people *with* the condition, as not having the condition). A low specificity means that the screening method results in many 'false positives' (i.e. it would identify many people without the condition as having the condition).

Higher *sensitivity* may be preferred for infectious disease control, to reduce the number of false negatives that could result in continued transmission of the disease. Higher *specificity* may be preferred for a screening programme where the subsequent diagnostic test for an outcome is very expensive or carries health risks, to avoid performing unnecessary procedures on many false positives.

Predictive values

From the individual's perspective, it is more useful to know the 'predictive value' of a screening method. The **positive predictive value** (PPV) is the likelihood of outcome based on the result, while the **negative predictive value** (NPV) is the likelihood of no outcome based on the result. For example, the PPV of mammography will tell a woman how likely it is that she truly has breast cancer if she has a positive mammogram, while the NPV will tell her how likely it is that she truly does not have breast cancer if she has a negative mammogram. Using the notation in Table 11.1, these are calculated as:

$$\text{Positive predictive value} = \frac{\textbf{Number of true positives}}{\textbf{Number tested positive}} = \frac{a}{a + b}$$

$$\text{Negative predictive value} = \frac{\textbf{Number of true negatives}}{\textbf{Number tested negative}} = \frac{d}{c + d}$$

Predictive values are determined by the sensitivity and specificity of the screening method. The higher the sensitivity, the less likely it is that an individual with a negative result will have the condition, so the greater the NPV of the method. The higher the specificity, the less likely it is that an individual with a positive result will actually not have the outcome, so the greater the PPV of the method.

Predictive values are also determined by the prevalence of the condition being screened for. Why? Remember that prevalence is calculated as the number of individuals who have the outcome, divided by the total number of individuals sampled. Consider that Table 11.1 has the same format as Table 3.1 (see Chapter 3), and think of the 'true condition' as the 'outcome' and the 'screening method result' as the 'exposure'. If you compare the formula for prevalence (Chapter 3) with those for PPV and NPV, you will see it effectively calculates the prevalence of the true condition among those 'exposed' and 'unexposed' to a positive result respectively.

Note, that the sensitivity and specificity of a screening method are independent of the prevalence of the condition in the population being screened. This is because sensitivity only relates to those who truly have the condition, while specificity only relates to those who truly do not have the condition. Therefore, in contrast to predictive values, neither measure considers the frequency (prevalence) of the true condition.

Ethical issues

In addition to assessing the validity of a screening method, the ethical consequences of screening must be evaluated. The risks of screening can be considered at both individual and population levels. An unwell person seeking medical help is willing to undergo a medical examination and associated tests in the hope of receiving a definitive diagnosis and appropriate treatment. However, a screening test is a preventive intervention applied to outwardly healthy individuals with no symptoms of the outcome.

It is therefore essential that the benefits of participating in screening outweigh the risks. It is an ethical responsibility to provide enough information for individuals to make an informed decision about whether or not to participate. While many screening methods present no risk, others have the potential to harm the participant (e.g. repeated exposure to X-ray radiation in mammography for breast cancer, or increased risk of miscarriage following an amniocentesis test to identify Down's syndrome pregnancies).

All screening methods will result in false negatives and false positives, either through low sensitivity or specificity, or because of human error. A false positive result can cause unnecessary anxiety while a false negative result can lead to a loss of confidence in medical intervention or a potential loss of life. An individual with a false negative result is provided with a false sense of security and may fail to recognize subsequent symptoms, resulting in poorer outcomes. Even a true positive result may increase anxiety, posing a risk to mental health or quality of life, while health and life insurance premiums may also increase.

Before introducing a national screening policy, any additional resource requirements must be planned for. Good quality control is essential to ensure correct functioning of a screening programme. Any variation in standards and criteria used to indicate further intervention may result in poor compliance, reducing the proportion of the population likely to benefit. Specialist equipment may be required. Staff may require additional training. Pre- and post-test counselling may be necessary. The incidence of the condition must be estimated to plan for the numbers requiring screening and the subsequent proportion needing further diagnostic tests or expensive treatments. It is unethical to screen if there will be insufficient facilities or effective treatments for those who need them.

Criteria for screening

The World Health Organization developed criteria for assessing the appropriateness of screening in 1968 (Wilson and Jungner 1968) that continue to be used today (see Table 11.2). Some of these criteria are context-specific and may differ from the point of view of the individual or community.

Using these criteria, we can evaluate whether or not to implement a screening programme. The three main themes to consider are: (1) relative burden of the condition; (2) feasibility of organizing a screening programme; and (3) potential effectiveness of a programme. An outcome that is rare but very serious and easily preventable may be worth screening for. For example, Phenylketonuria, a congenitally acquired inability to metabolize the amino acid phenylalanine, is a rare disease. If undetected, it leads to serious mental retardation. A highly sensitive and specific screening test, performed on a blood sample taken from a prick in the heel of a newborn, can identify babies who have this condition. A diet low in phenylalanine can then effectively prevent development of mental retardation in these children.

Table 11.2 List of ten WHO criteria for assessing the appropriateness of screening

Focus	Criterion
Condition:	The condition being screened for should be an important health problem The natural history of the condition should be well understood There should be a recognizable latent or early stage
Method:	There should be a suitable method for detection The screening method should be acceptable to the population
Treatment:	There should be an accepted treatment for those with the condition
Programme:	There should be an agreed policy on who to treat Facilities for diagnosis and treatment should be available The costs of detection should be balanced in relation to overall healthcare spending Screening should be ongoing and not one-off

Source: Ilona Carneiro, using data from Wilson and Jungner (1968).

The relative burden of the condition compared with other health problems should justify the expense of a screening programme in relation to the resources available. However wealthy a society is, there will always be finite resources available for healthcare. The resource costs of a screening programme need to be balanced with the cost-savings of treating fewer patients identified at a later stage with an advanced outcome. The feasibility of organizing a screening programme will depend on:

1 systems for identifying and contacting individuals (e.g. general practioner's lists, mother and child health clinics, schools);
2 compliance levels (e.g. colonoscopy to detect colon cancer is invasive, uncomfortable and may not be acceptable to sufficient individuals);
3 whether facilities are in place for more extensive diagnostic tests if needed (e.g. a mammography campaign will result in a greater than usual referral for breast biopsies);
4 availability of resources for increased treatment (e.g. screening for cholesterol will result in increased demand for cholesterol-lowering drugs).

Measuring effectiveness

The potential effectiveness of a programme to reduce the frequency of a condition is hard to measure and often subject to various biases. **Selection bias** occurs because those who participate in screening programmes often differ from those who do not. Women who are at high risk of breast cancer because of family history may be more likely to attend for mammography. By contrast, women at low risk of cervical cancer appear to be more likely to accept an invitation for a cervical smear test.

Lead-time bias can occur when screening identifies an outcome earlier than it would otherwise have been identified, but has no effect on the outcome. For example, a disease that would otherwise be diagnosed at 60 years when symptoms arise might be detected by screening Test A at 55 years and by Test B at 50 years (see Figure 11.3). Even without medical intervention, it may appear that Test A prolongs survival for five years and Test B for ten years, whereas this is a consequence of earlier detection. This effect must be considered when evaluating the results of a screening method, by using outcome measures other than survival time.

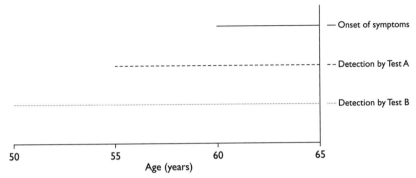

Figure 11.3 Lead-time bias effect for a disease with onset at 50 years and death at 65 years

Source: Ilona Carneiro, modified from Bailey et al. (2005).

Length-time bias can occur for outcomes that take longer to develop to a stage where they threaten health (i.e. longer **asymptomatic** period). For example, slower-growing breast cancer tumours are more likely to be detected by screening prior to the development of symptoms than faster-growing tumours. However, slower-growing tumours may also be less aggressive and associated with a better **prognosis**, leading to an over-estimate of the screening success. Consider a population of 100 people with cancer: 20 have slower-growing tumours and all are detected by screening, 80 have faster-growing tumours only half (40) of which are detected by screening before they develop symptoms. If all of the slower-growing tumours and none of the faster-growing tumours respond to subsequent treatment, we would calculate the success of screening as 20 ÷ (20 + 40) = 33%. However, the true success should be measured over all those detected and un-detected by the screening, as 20 ÷ 100 = 20%.

It is difficult to identify appropriate study designs to evaluate screening programmes because of these biases. Table 11.3 summarizes potential study designs and the key biases that may arise.

Table 11.3 Comparison of methods and biases of study designs for evaluating screening methods

Study type	Method	Potential biases
Cohort	Compares time to adverse outcome in screen-detected and non-screen-detected cases	Lead-time bias Length-time bias
Case control	Compares screening history of cases with age-matched controls	Selection bias Information bias
Non-randomized trial	Compares outcome using a historical or neighbourhood comparison group	Selection bias
Randomized-controlled trial	Compares outcome between individuals randomly allocated to screening or control groups	Information bias Misclassification bias

Source: Ilona Carneiro, adapted from Bailey et al. (2005).

A randomized-controlled trial (RCT) is the best method for evaluation (see Chapter 10), as the effects of lead-time, length-time and selection biases are balanced by random allocation. However, it may not be appropriate to use an RCT for screening if the screening method has already been introduced into a population or if the population perceives the screening as beneficial (even if unproven). It is unethical to undertake a 'blind' trial where participants receive placebo screening, as those given a false-negative result from placebo-screening may be less likely to notice symptom development and delay treatment-seeking. If those responsible for subsequent patient care are aware of the trial and subject allocation, this may affect their knowledge, recognition of subsequent symptoms, and attribution of cause in the case of death (observer bias). There may be a risk of 'contamination' if awareness of a screening programme leads subjects in the control (non-screened) group to seek-out screening, which may lead to differential misclassification of exposure to screening. As many of the conditions that would be screened for are relatively rare, large sample sizes would be necessary to detect a significant effect.

Activity 11.2

In a hypothetical study, 1,000 patients attending a hospital general outpatient department were tested for diabetes using the following two tests:

- fasting blood sugar (FBS)
- glucose tolerance test (GTT).

The 100 patients with a positive GTT were classified as true cases of diabetes. Of 140 patients with an FBS of at least 6 mmol/l (the cut-off point to distinguish people who have diabetes from those who do not), only 98 were true cases of diabetes (i.e. only 98 also had a positive GTT).

1 What are the sensitivity, specificity, and positive and negative predictive values of the FBS test in this study population? You may find it useful to create a 2×2 table of the information given.
2 When the cut-off point for the FBS was raised to 7 mmol/l, the sensitivity of the test decreased to 95% while specificity increased to 98%. Create a new 2×2 table using this new cut-off and calculate:
    (a) the positive predictive value of FBS in the study population;
    (b) the proportion of diabetics given a false negative FBS result.

3 In a subsequent community survey to screen for diabetes, of 1,000 people surveyed, 40 had a positive GTT and were classified as true cases of diabetes. Using a cut-off value of 6 mmol/l the FBS had a sensitivity of 97.5% and specificity of 95%. What is the positive predictive value of FBS in this survey and why is it different from that observed in the hospital-based study?

4 If the FBS cut-off point is increased to 7.5 mmol/l, the sensitivity is 90% and the specificity is 99% for diagnosing diabetes in the community.
    If you were to fix the cut-off point of FBS for a survey in your community would you select 6 mmol/l or 7.5 mmol/l? Give reasons for your answer.

Targeting high-risk individuals

When there are appropriate methods to identify individuals at high risk of an outcome (e.g. screening), it may be tempting to target interventions at 'high-risk' individuals rather than a whole community. This is a more of clinically oriented approach to prevention. The focus on the individual is sometimes perceived as easier to promote since the impact of high-risk exposure is more apparent to those at greatest risk, so they may be more likely to comply and therefore benefit from an intervention. Another benefit of the high-risk approach is that it fits with society's perception of the role of medical intervention (i.e. focusing on needy individuals, rather than aiming to change the behaviour of the whole population to achieve general health gains).

The general population would be unlikely to consent to testing for sexually transmitted infections (STIs) to stop an increasing incidence of STIs, expecting such screening to be targeted at those who practice 'risky' sexual behaviours (e.g. multiple sexual partners, unprotected sex). Similarly, it would not be cost-effective to provide routine mammograms to women under 30 years of age, given that the main burden of breast cancer is in women over 50 years of age and mammograms are costly.

However, when assessing whether an individual is in a high-risk group, definitions or screening methods should be accurate. Labelling individuals as 'high-risk' can cause unnecessary anxiety in healthy individuals and may even be stigmatizing. Criteria should be standardized to prevent a blurring of categories (e.g. being slightly overweight can merge with being more overweight which can merge with being labelled 'obese').

Another limitation of this approach is that it does not always seek to change the circumstances that encourage exposure to a known risk factor (i.e. it does not address the root-causes of risky exposures). For example, vaccination of people at risk of a water-borne disease without efforts to improve the quality of the local water supply, or the use of cholesterol-lowering drugs rather than improving diet, are temporary solutions. This may also shift the burden of responsibility (and 'guilt') to high-risk individuals or groups, while failing to recognize the role of external influences such as economics and advertising, which ultimately affect the wider population.

The high-risk approach may not be able to predict the individual impact of an intervention as levels of risk and outcome will vary within risk groups. Therefore, individuals are unable to make an informed decision about whether to comply. It may also be argued that the targeted approach is exclusive, and that all individuals should have access to interventions that improve general health. Finally, targeting high-risk groups may be more expensive, often requiring mass screening to identify at-risk individuals.

The prevention paradox and the population approach

Another problem with targeting those at highest risk occurs when those individuals are only a small proportion of the total population at risk. In such circumstances, a large risk reduction among a few high-risk individuals may not have any population-level impact on an outcome, while a slight risk reduction among many people may have a large impact at the population level. This is known as the **prevention paradox**.

For example, a number of risk factors have been identified for heart attack (myocardial infarction or MI), including smoking, raised blood pressure, high cholesterol and psychosocial stress. The risk of MI increases with the number of risk factors to which an individual is exposed. However, a prevention strategy that focused on those individuals with elevated risk factors (see Table 11.4), would reach just 15% of men of whom only 9% would subsequently develop a MI (i.e. 91% of those targeted would not experience MI). Targeting individuals with elevated risk factors *and* signs of early heart disease whose risk of MI is much greater (22%), would prevent just 11% of all MIs.

As 61% of MIs occur in men who are not at high-risk, primary prevention of MI should be directed at the whole population. If a population-wide strategy was put into place and all men over a certain age modified their behaviour slightly, the public health

Table 11.4 Distribution of myocardial infarction (MI) by high-risk group

Risk group	Total (% under study)	Developed MI (% of sub-group)	Percentage of MI cases (n = 403)
All men under study	8,147 (100)	245 (4)	61
Elevated risk factors	1,222 (15)	115 (9)	29
Elevated risk factors and evidence of early disease	199 (2)	43 (22)	11

Source: Ilona Carneiro, adapted from Heller et al. (1984) and Rose (1992).

benefit could be considerable. This illustrates the fact that targeting high-risk groups may not be appropriate in a situation where a small risk affects a large proportion of the population and will therefore generate a large number of cases.

The prevention paradox can be applied to individuals who modify their behaviour to reduce exposure to known risk factors in the hope of avoiding an outcome. As most outcomes are rare, many individuals who adopt a certain lifestyle or behaviour designed to reduce their risk of adverse outcome will not benefit directly (because they would never have developed the outcome), while a few individuals will benefit greatly (because they would otherwise have developed the outcome). The greatest public benefit will therefore often come from applying a preventive intervention to the whole population.

Rose (1992) argued that it is not only the extreme cases that require attention, but also the much larger proportion of people with milder features of an outcome. In addition, individuals are not always simply exposed or not exposed to a risk factor, but may be exposed to varying degrees. For a risk factor with a 'normal' population distribution (i.e. very few people are highly exposed, very few people are not exposed, and the majority are somewhat exposed to the risk factor), it makes more sense to reduce everyone's exposure rather than targeting the very few at highest risk.

Choosing the appropriate approach

To decide whether to take an individual or population approach to preventive intervention, we must consider the characteristics of the intervention. Some preventive measures can only be implemented on a mass scale (e.g. fluoridation of water to prevent tooth decay, environmental legislation to control air pollution). However, for outcomes where the greatest burden is known to be concentrated among high-risk individuals, it may be more appropriate to target high-risk groups rather than the whole population, if we can adequately identify those at high risk. Alternatively, there may be benefits to using both approaches together. For example, in HIV prevention, health education messages on safer sex practices are aimed at the whole population, while sex-workers and drug-users may be targeted for HIV-screening, and given improved access to condoms and disposable needles respectively.

If we have sufficient information on the prevalence of risk factors and incidence of outcome, we can calculate the population-attributable fraction for a risk factor (see Chapter 3) and compare the proportion of cases that could be prevented by using either the population or high-risk approach. The appropriate approach also depends on whether the intervention will be implemented in the community, within hospitals or in a primary healthcare setting.

Activity 11.3

Figure 11.4 contrasts population distributions of serum cholesterol in Japan and Finland. Elevated serum cholesterol is a risk factor for coronary heart disease.

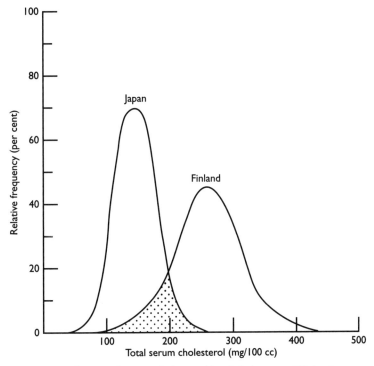

Figure 11.4 Population distribution of serum cholesterol levels in Japan and Finland
Source: Rose (1992).

1 Describe what Figure 11.4 shows.
2 List some potential explanations for the difference in serum cholesterol distribution between these populations.
3 Would you choose a population or high-risk prevention strategy to reduce the risk of coronary heart disease in the Finnish population? Give reasons for your answer.

Activity 11.4

1 You are responsible for developing a public health strategy to reduce fatal injuries as the result of road traffic crashes. Describe at which level of prevention each of the following interventions could be involved.
   (a) Car seat-belt restraints.
   (b) Driving speed limits.
   (c) Paramedic pre-hospital care at the crash site.

Activity 11.5

1 Human papilloma virus (HPV) has been identified as a necessary cause of cervical cancer, although it is not a sufficient cause and the majority of those infected do not develop cervical cancer. A programme of routine vaccination of adolescent girls against HPV is to be conducted in country X, where the prevalence of HPV among women is 10% and the incidence of cervical cancer is 10 per 100,000 women per year. Is this an example of the 'prevention paradox'? Explain your answer.

Conclusion

In this chapter you have learned about different prevention strategies (primary, secondary, tertiary) relating to intervention stage and dose–response relationship. As screening is key in secondary prevention, you learned statistical methods for evaluating screening methods (i.e. sensitivity, specificity, and predictive values) and evaluation of a screening programme using WHO criteria. Public health approaches may be targeted or general, depending on risk distribution, relative outcome burden in the population, and intervention delivery method. While a population approach can be more effective given the 'prevention paradox', a combination of both approaches is often most powerful.

References

Bailey L, Vardulaki K, Langham J and Chandramohan D (2005) *Introduction to Epidemiology*. Maidenhead: Open University Press.
Heller RF, Chinn S, Pedoe HD and Rose G (1984) How well can we predict coronary heart disease? Findings in the United Kingdom Heart Disease Prevention Project. *British Medical Journal (Clin Res Ed)* 288: 1409–11.
Rose G (1992) *The Strategy of Preventive Medicine*. Oxford: Oxford University Press.
Wilson JM and Jungner YG (1968) *Principles and Practice of Screening for Disease. Public Health Papers*. Geneva: World Health Organization.

Feedback for activities

Activity 11.1

1 Your answers should be similar to the following:
  (a) Exposure increases without adverse outcome until a particular level is reached, after which the risk of outcome increases rapidly. It would be most appropriate to target preventive interventions to those at high risk of exposure.

   For example, an increase in intra-ocular (inside the eye) pressure is not dangerous until it exceeds certain levels. Above these levels the incidence of glaucoma (damage to the optic nerve affecting vision and eventually leading to blindness) rises rapidly. It is therefore desirable to keep intra-ocular pressure under the threshold, but there is no benefit to be gained in further reducing it.

   Note, however, that the definition of a threshold level beyond which adverse effects appear is derived from population data. At an individual level, there may be some people with adverse outcomes below the threshold, while others continue to be healthy despite being above the threshold.

(b) There is a linear relationship between the exposure and outcome. The greater the exposure, the greater the risk, even at very low exposure levels. Shifting the whole population exposure towards lower levels will bring beneficial effects and is the most appropriate public health objective.

For example, there is an increased risk of lung cancer even with the small amounts of tobacco smoke associated with passive smoking. There is no safe level of exposure to tobacco smoke, but removing all exposure would be very difficult. Health promotion activities and legislation at the population level are the best way to achieve the large change in behaviour necessary to reduce population exposure.

(c) The risk of outcome increases with exposure, but the slope is shallow at lower exposure and increases more rapidly at higher exposures. If a large proportion of the outcome is due to those at higher exposure, then it would be appropriate to target preventive interventions to those at high risk. However, if the majority of outcome is due to those at lower exposure (because few individuals have a high exposure), then it would be more appropriate to shift the whole population towards a reduced exposure.

This curved exposure to outcome relationship is usually a more accurate description than the oversimplified linear relationship above. For example, in osteoporosis, the bone mineral density (BMD) is reduced, resulting in fractures, which can be prevented with appropriate medication. The risk of hip fracture increases gradually with declining BMD until about 700–800 mg/cm^2 below which the risk increases more rapidly. The relative benefit of bone-density X-ray scans depends on the distribution of BMD in the population, and this distribution shifts with age. The benefit of bone-density scans is greater in post-menopausal women in whom the likelihood of low BMD is greater.

(d) This relationship is more complex, showing a wide range of exposure during which there is no increased risk of outcome, with increased risk of outcome at very low and very high exposure. This fits the common belief that 'moderation is good and extremes are bad'. For this dose–response pattern, there are inherent problems in shifting the entire population too far in either direction, and either a targeted approach or a complex intervention for the whole population is required.

For example, for a given body size, there is a wide range of weight that carries no increased risk of adverse outcome. At the extremes of low weight and high weight, however, there may be associated health hazards. A policy that aims to decrease body-weight for the entire population might inadvertently shift some low weight people into the extremely underweight category associated with increased mortality. The health promotion messages therefore need to be more sophisticated and complex.

Activity 11.2

1 Your 2×2 table of FBS test by true diabetes (GTT test) should look like Table 11.5.

Explanation of rationale:

Of the total 1,000 patients tested, 100 had a positive GTT (i.e. diabetic), therefore 1,000 – 100 = 900 had a negative GTT (i.e. not diabetic). Of the 1,000, 140 had a positive FBS, therefore 1,000 – 140 = 860 had a negative FBS. Of the 140 positive FBS, 98 were also

Table 11.5 FBS test results (cut-off 6 mmol/l) by true diabetes (GTT test) status

True diabetes (GTT)			
Test results (FBS)	Diabetic	Not diabetic	Total
Positive	98	42	140
Negative	2	858	860
Total	100	900	1,000

Source: Bailey et al. (2005).

positive for GTT (diabetic), therefore 140 − 98 = 42 were negative for GTT (not diabetic).

The sensitivity of FBS is the number of true positives detected by the test, divided by the total of number of diabetics (GTT positive): 98 ÷ 100 = 0.98 or 98%

The specificity of FBS is the number of true negatives detected by the test, divided by the total number not diabetic (GTT negative): 858 ÷ 900 = 0.95 or 95%

The positive predictive value of FBS is the number of true positives divided by the total detected positive by the test: 98 ÷ 140 = 0.70 or 70%

The negative predictive value of FBS is the number of true negatives divided by the total detected negative by the test: 858 ÷ 860 = 0.998 or 99.8%

2 The new 2*2 table using the 7 mmol/l cut-off should look like Table 11.6.

Table 11.6 FBS test results (cut-off 7 mmol/l) by true diabetes (GTT test) status

True diabetes (GTT)			
Test results (FBS)	Diabetic	Not diabetic	Total
Positive	95	18	113
Negative	5	882	887
Total	100	900	1,000

Source: Bailey et al. (2005).

Explanation of rationale:

We know that the number of diabetics was 100, and the number not diabetic was 900. If the sensitivity of the test decreased to 95%, this means that 0.95 × 100 = 95 of the diabetics (GTT positive) were diagnosed positive using the new FBS cut-off, and the remaining 5 diabetics were diagnosed as negative by FBS. If the specificity increased to 98%, it means that 0.98 × 900 = 882 of those not diabetic were diagnosed as negative using the new FBS cut-off, and 900 − 882 = 18 of those not diabetic were diagnosed as positive by FBS.

(a) The positive predictive value of FBS using the new cut-off is 95 ÷ 113 = 0.84 or 84%

(b) The proportion of false negatives with FBS is 5 ÷ 100 = 0.05 or 5%.
    Alternatively, it can be calculated directly from knowledge of the sensitivity only as: 1 − sensitivity = 1 − 0.95 = 0.05 or 5%.

3 As before, you should have started by setting up a 2×2 table as shown in Table 11.7.

Table 11.7 FBS test results (cut-off 6 mmol/l) by true diabetes (GTT test) status

True diabetes (GTT)			
Test results (FBS)	Diabetic	Not diabetic	Total
Positive	39	48	87
Negative	1	912	913
Total	40	960	1,000

Source: Bailey et al. (2005).

Explanation of rationale:

If 40 were truly diabetic, then 1,000 − 40 = 960 were not diabetic using GTT. If FBS had 97.5% sensitivity, then 0.975 × 40 = 39 diabetics were detected as positive by the FBS test, and 40 − 39 = 1 diabetic was detected as negative by FBS. If FBS had 95% specificity, then 0.95 × 960 = 912 of those not diabetic were detected as negative by the FBS test, and 960 − 912 = 48 of those not diabetic were detected as positive by FBS.

The positive predictive value of FBS is the number of true positives divided by the total detected positive by the test: 39 ÷ 87 = 0.45 or 45%.

Although the sensitivity and specificity of the FBS using a cut-off 6 mmol/l were almost the same in the hospital-based and community surveys, there is marked reduction in the positive predictive value of FBS in the community survey. This is because the prevalence of diabetes in the hospital population was higher (100 ÷ 1,000 = 10%) than in the community (40 ÷ 1,000 = 4%).

4 You should have chosen 6 mmol/l as an appropriate cut-off point for FBS in the community, because the sensitivity is higher at 6 mmol/l (97.5%) than at 7.5 mmol/l (90%), so that we detect a greater proportion of diabetics. It is better to have fewer false negative results (2% vs. 10%), as there are effective treatments for diabetes that can effectively prevent later complications so that timely intervention matters.

This is preferable to a higher specificity with fewer false positives, as the implications of false positives for an outcome such as diabetes are not very severe. The physical and psychological stress following a false positive test for diabetes is minimal since further diagnostic tests (e.g. GTT) are available to refute the diagnosis.

Activity 11.3

1 The Japanese distribution curve is taller with a narrow spread, and the majority of samples around 150mg/100cc. This suggests that most of the Japanese population presents with a lower level of cholesterol and that there is little variation. The Finnish distribution curve is shorter with a wider spread, and the majority of samples around 250mg/100cc. This suggests that the Finnish population has a higher average serum cholesterol level with more variation. While the two distributions do overlap, the majority of the Finnish population have higher levels of cholesterol than the Japanese population.

2 When there are major differences between populations, as shown in Figure 11.4, it suggests that some community-level factor is determining the difference. There may

be genetic, behavioural (e.g. diet), or environmental differences between the populations that may be addressed as part of any prevention strategy.

3 A population approach would be appropriate if the aim is to shift the whole Finnish distribution curve towards lower cholesterol levels, making it more similar to the Japanese distribution. A high-risk approach would be appropriate if the aim is to reduce cholesterol levels only in those with extremely high values.

In deciding which approach would have a greater public health impact, you would need to know the shape of the relationship between cholesterol level and risk of coronary heart disease.

If there are behavioural or environmental differences, it may be possible to shift the entire distribution in a healthier direction with a population-level prevention strategy if appropriate policies are adopted. A moderate change by the whole population might greatly reduce the number of people with the most extreme cholesterol levels. Thus, while many individuals might each receive a small benefit, the total benefit to the whole population may still be larger than with a targeted approach.

Activity 11.4

The process of outcome development can be simply outlined as: (i) road traffic crash, (ii) serious injury, (iii) death. The level of prevention for each intervention can be explained as:

(a) Secondary prevention because car seat-belt restraints act to reduce injury in case of a crash

(b) Primary prevention because driving speed limits aim to reduce road traffic crashes from occurring

(c) Tertiary prevention because on-site medical care may reduce the risk of death from serious injuries.

Activity 11.5

Yes, this is an example of the prevention paradox, as many women will receive the intervention, but only a small proportion of these will benefit. We can estimate that 90% of those to be vaccinated would not have contracted HPV anyway, and the majority of those who might have contracted HPV would not have then developed cervical cancer. Therefore, at an individual level, the risk reduction is small. However, at a population level, the risk reduction is great, as HPV is one of the leading causes of cancer mortality.

Surveillance, monitoring and evaluation | 12

Overview

In earlier chapters, you learned how to conduct epidemiological research studies and how to interpret their results. In the previous chapter, you considered different approaches to preventive interventions. In this chapter, you will be introduced to public health surveillance systems and methods for monitoring and evaluating public health programmes. Many of the research methods you have learned can be adapted for use under routine conditions, so that public health may continue to be evidence-based even after research has been completed.

Learning objectives

When you have completed this chapter you should be able to:

- describe the purpose and types of public health surveillance, and the importance of registries and notifiable diseases in surveillance
- identify indicators that may be used for evaluating public health programmes
- discuss the role of epidemiological data in informing public health policy and practice.

Health information systems

The health information system (HIS) of a country aims to integrate the collection, analysis and reporting of data on health outcomes, to provide evidence for improving health services and ultimately the population's health. This may include population-based data, i.e. censuses and vital registration systems (discussed in Chapter 6), routinely collected health facility data and surveillance of notifiable diseases and registries. Repeated cross-sectional surveys for specific diseases may also be carried out as part of monitoring a population's health.

Use of routinely collected data

Regular, systematic and accurate reporting of health outcomes allows us to determine the usual 'baseline' outcome frequency in a population, and to look at variations between populations and over time. The prevalence of known risk factors for adverse health outcomes, such as smoking and alcohol consumption, may also be monitored using household health surveys to review population behaviours over time. For example, the Behavioral Risk Factor Surveillance System in the USA uses telephone surveys of randomly sampled adults to obtain such data, while information on occupational risks may come from employer records.

Changes in frequency over time may be described as secular or seasonal. A *secular trend* refers to a change that is expected to be sustained over a long period of time. For example, Figure 12.1 shows a decline in syphilis among men and women in the USA between 1993 and 1998, but a subsequent increase among men since 2000. Changes in time can indicate that public health efforts are working, or alert the health system to a growing health danger.

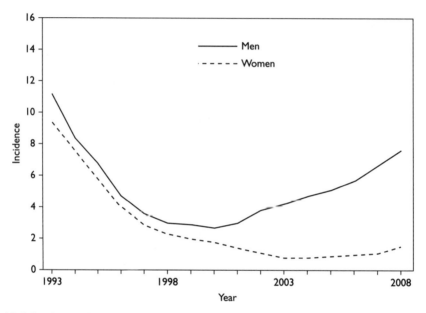

Figure 12.1 Incidence of notified syphilis cases in the USA per 100,000 population by gender and year
Source: Centers for Disease Control and Prevention (2010).

Other explanations for observed changes over time may be related to a change in the way data are collected or in the case definition. Such changes need to be documented and considered when interpreting a change in the expected incidence of an outcome. Figure 12.2 shows how an expansion of the case definition for AIDS in the USA in 1993 led to an artificial increase in the numbers of cases reported. Changes may also be due to awareness. For example, an examining doctor may be more likely to diagnose a particular outcome after a real or suspected outbreak, leading to *case-ascertainment bias* and an apparent increase in incidence.

Seasonal trends in frequency refer to changes that occur periodically, usually with a defined time cycle. Many childhood infections to which immunity is acquired show cycles of two to three years length. Many outcomes show a seasonal (i.e. intra-annual) variation that is related to changes in weather (e.g. vector-borne disease, meningitis). For example, cardiac mortality rates tend to increase during colder months in both the northern and southern hemispheres. Expected seasonal variation must be incorporated into any estimates of baseline incidence, for example to distinguish seasonal peaks from the start of an epidemic (e.g. influenza).

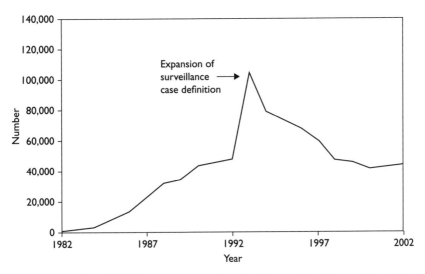

Figure 12.2 Total number of AIDS cases reported to the Centers for Disease Control in the USA between 1982 and 2002

Source: Centers for Disease Control and Prevention (2004).

Once baseline and normal variations are known, unusual changes can be more easily detected, highlighting an **outbreak** or the emergence of a new health problem. A sudden increase in the incidence of measles in a population, for example, can be investigated together with possible explanations (e.g. a decline in vaccination coverage).

Routine data can be compared between different populations, if they share the same demographic structure, or if this has been adjusted for using standardization methods (see Chapter 6). Data on different geographic areas within a country, urban or rural residence, socio-economic status, ethnicity and religion may be collected to enable inequalities in health outcomes and the use of healthcare to be investigated. The use of geographical information systems enables data to be mapped, highlighting focus areas for attention. For example, Figure 12.3 shows the prevalence of obesity by county in the USA in 2007, enabling further epidemiological research and preventive health promotion to be more accurately targeted.

Population-based data

In Chapter 6, you learned about censuses and vital registration to collect demographic data. We will review the uses of these routine data sources for monitoring a population's health.

Vital registration collects data on all registered births and deaths, providing data on population denominators, demographic structure, birth and mortality rates, and key health indicators. Registration of births may include information on health-related conditions, such as length of gestation, birthweight and congenital malformations. Mortality data can be used as an indicator of the incidence of specific outcomes, and of the population's health overall. These data can be used for planning health services, and may be compared between populations and monitored over time to identify issues of

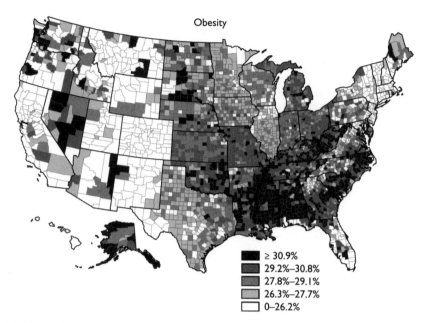

Figure 12.3 Age-adjusted percentage of adults ≥ 20 years old who were obese in the USA in 2007
Source: Centers for Disease Control and Prevention (2009).

concern. In countries with poor vital registration systems this information is obtained from sample vital registration or population censuses (see Chapter 6).

Population censuses aim to collect data on the age, gender, ethnicity, religion, occupation, etc. of all residents. These data are useful to assist the planning and allocation of health service resources and policy-making. Rigorous methods and quality control must be used to avoid information bias (e.g. exaggeration of sub-national population if it is perceived that government services are linked population size). There will be some *selection bias* as population subgroups, such as the homeless and migrant workers, will be under-represented. Statistical methods are used to estimate the data for intervening years between census surveys, and to make projections about future trends.

Public health surveillance

Public health **surveillance** is the monitoring of health in a given population over time. In Chapter 1, you saw an early example of this through John Snow's monitoring of the distribution of cholera-related deaths temporally (i.e. over time) and spatially (i.e. by geographic area). It enabled him to identify a pattern, and to generate and test his hypotheses on drinking water as the source of the epidemic. Modern surveillance systems also aim to provide timely information on which to base public health decisions, and for the planning, implementation, and evaluation of public health policies and practices.

Surveillance can detect and verify the emergence of health hazards such as infectious disease outbreaks, or more gradual increases in cause-specific deaths over time that may indicate changes in exposure to a risk factor. This enables initiation of an appropriate public health response to minimize any adverse impact on the health of a population.

A reporting framework is necessary for the systematic collection, analysis, interpretation and dissemination of health data. While these exist for specified infectious and chronic diseases, for many outcomes there is no specific surveillance system in place.

The development of a surveillance system requires clear objectives and the use of strict criteria with which to identify and classify disease. A clear case definition is vital to ensure accurate data are collected and detection is usually based on clinical findings, laboratory results to confirm a diagnosis, and epidemiological data describing the time, place and type of individuals affected. Standardized reporting methods are essential if authorities are to have confidence in the data collected.

However, many factors can affect data quality. Large numbers of people are usually responsible for surveillance data collection across many sites. Without the opportunity for specific training, the validity of data may suffer. Feeding-back data to the individuals collecting it can motivate them to ensure data are of a high standard. Motivation to record data systematically may also be influenced by perception of whether the capacity and infrastructure exist to elicit an appropriate public health response.

Types of surveillance

Surveillance systems may be passive or active. **Passive surveillance** is the detection of cases when they seek healthcare. Responsibility for reporting is placed on the health service provider (e.g. doctor, laboratory, health centre, hospital), which will routinely collect data on the numbers, basic demographics and diagnoses of patients seen. Practitioners may also report to registries that centralize data on specific chronic conditions (e.g. cancers). Passive surveillance also includes the use of certified death data to monitor cause-specific mortality (see Chapter 6).

Active surveillance involves case-finding using methods such as reviews of clinical records or community health surveys. Active surveillance is costly and labour-intensive, and is not usually used for routine surveillance unless (a) there is a need to monitor the emergence or elimination of a new disease, or (b) when cases may not be accessing the formal healthcare infrastructure.

Health facility data

Public hospitals and clinics generally collect data on outpatient and inpatient attendance, together with basic patient demographics and diagnoses, which is collated and reported to a central body. Health facility data cannot be used to estimate the true incidence of an outcome in the population, because many factors will influence whether or not an individual attends a health facility. For example, some individuals may seek care from the private, voluntary, or informal sectors (e.g. traditional healers, medication sellers), and they would not be included in estimates of incidence calculated from public hospital data. Access to healthcare also varies geographically and with socio-economics.

These data may still be used to monitor the healthcare needs of a population, and as an indicator of what may be occurring in the population, as long as we are aware of their biases. For example, an unexpected increase in patients attending with influenza may suggest the start of an epidemic that requires more comprehensive population-based surveillance and health advice. In low-income settings, where the health services are already overloaded, there may be minimal record keeping and the data may not be an accurate reflection of the situation.

While many effective surveillance systems function around the world, the proportion of outcomes recorded and reported will vary and surveillance is unlikely to capture all cases. Population incidence calculated from routine surveillance is therefore likely to underestimate the true incidence in the community.

Registry data

A registry is a systematic collection of data about every patient with a particular diagnosis, condition or procedure (e.g. cancer, artificial joints). Registries allow the monitoring of individual patients over time and may be used to coordinate recall of patients to attend for regular check-ups and reviews of medication. Information is collected on various factors including basic demographics, patient history, diagnosis, treatment and health status. Data may come from general practitioners, treatment facilities, hospitals or death certificates.

Registers are also used for surveillance. In the UK, the National Congenital Anomaly System (NCAS) was established in 1964 in response to the thalidomide tragedy. Thalidomide was licensed for use by pregnant women as a medication to reduce nausea but was subsequently found to cause limb malformations in the unborn child. The NCAS was set up to detect new hazards and help prevent a similar tragedy. Although the main purpose of the NCAS is surveillance, it also provides valuable birth prevalence data.

Another example comes from Australia's Northern Territory, which reports the highest published incidence of acute rheumatic fever (ARF) in the world among its Aboriginal population. Since recurrent cases of ARF lead to cumulative heart valve damage, ARF is a significant cause of cardiovascular morbidity and mortality for these communities. Since 1997, a rheumatic heart disease control programme has established a computerized registry of all known or suspected cases of ARF or rheumatic heart disease within the region. The registry is used to improve patient care, particularly secondary prevention, by establishing a reminder system for monthly penicillin injections and other clinical follow-up by the primary care system, and to organize and conduct education programmes.

Registries can be used to monitor outcome incidence, prevalence and patient survival over time. Analysis of registry data can be used to evaluate the effectiveness of screening programmes, other preventive interventions, treatments or surgical procedures using cohort study designs. Healthcare providers may also collect information to monitor the quality of care (e.g. treatment waiting times, average length of stay in hospital). By analysing registry data on previous patients, healthcare providers can inform patients, and plan, monitor and improve their services. Registry data can also be analysed in ecological studies to compare populations using standardized rates (see Chapter 6) and to develop hypotheses on possible disease causation by considering patient characteristics and environmental exposures.

Infectious disease surveillance

Many countries have systems in place for monitoring certain **notifiable diseases** (e.g. cholera, tuberculosis, yellow fever) through compulsory (i.e. legally enforced) reporting. The health service provider must keep detailed records and notify a central public health agency of each notifiable case diagnosed. Data on notifiable diseases are then collated and analysed by public health agencies (e.g. Health Protection Agency in the UK, Centers for Disease Control and Prevention in the USA).

Notification rates will depend primarily on whether an affected individual seeks medical advice. In some communities, healthcare providers may be difficult to access or patients may be unaware of their condition and not seek help. The infrastructure may not exist to record data of sufficient quality and to communicate that data.

The list of notifiable diseases varies between countries, but the majority are infectious. If the infection is not **endemic** to a country, notification aims to identify importations and stop local transmission. If the infection is endemic, notification enables monitoring for early detection of, and rapid response to, an outbreak (see Figure 12.4). However, public health agencies need resources and infrastructure to act rapidly on the information they receive, if they are to successfully stop or slow the spread of a disease.

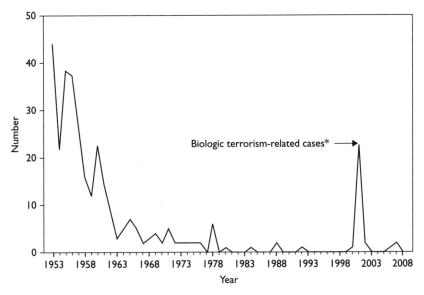

Figure 12.4 Number of cases of anthrax notified by year in the USA (1953–2008)

Source: Centers for Disease Control and Prevention (2010).

An example of the utility of surveillance for disease control is the use of epidemic-warning systems in the malaria epidemic-prone highlands of Africa (Jones et al. 2008). If routine data on the incidence of clinical malaria cases attending a health facility are collected and analysed in a timely manner, abnormal patterns can be identified early in the epidemic. This allows for implementation of appropriate preventive measures, such as indoor-residual spraying of houses with insecticide, which may avert a major epidemic. Previously, the delays inherent in collating paper-based clinic records and summarizing data for each area resulted in data reaching the malaria control programme too late to be of use. Knowing this, clinic staff had no incentive to ensure that data were rigorously recorded. The introduction of computer databases to enter and summarize data, and appropriate training, has improved the accuracy and utility of the surveillance system. Data can be rapidly fed back to clinic staff, and the malaria control programme, which can take action as necessary.

Sentinel surveillance is the collection and analysis of data by designated institutions selected for their geographic location, disease specialization, and ability to accurately diagnose and report high quality data. It involves the identification of health providers and diagnostic facilities with sufficient capacity to participate in a reporting network. Sentinel surveillance may be appropriate when costly diagnostic tests are involved. For example, taking throat-swabs from patients with flu-like symptoms to obtain a laboratory diagnosis of influenza in the UK, or monitoring the spread of anti-malarial drug resistance across Africa. In low-income countries, this may require an initial investment of appropriate training and resources to develop a functioning network.

Outbreak response

The Global Polio Eradication Initiative has worked to strengthen surveillance of polio and reporting systems in low-income countries. As the programme nears its target, the numbers of cases of paralytic poliomyelitis decline, and detection of circulating wild poliovirus becomes harder. In countries that have already locally **eliminated** the disease, there is a risk that an importation of polio virus could lead to the re-establishment of local transmission. Consequently, surveillance is the key to successful **eradication**. While acute poliomyelitis is a notifiable disease, those countries without sufficient infrastructure may rely on reporting of all acute flaccid paralysis cases followed by a laboratory diagnosis. The global programme assesses how effectively a country's surveillance systems are functioning though a network of sentinel sites. Information on cases detected, importations and local outbreaks is analysed and shared to enable a rapid response using targeted vaccination.

The World Health Organization (WHO) coordinates a number of surveillance strategies around the world and aims to strengthen the capacity of countries to conduct effective surveillance. The International Health Regulations (2005), implemented since 2007, outline 'global rules to enhance national, regional and global public health security' that are legally binding for all member states (World Health Organization 2011b). These regulations require countries to strengthen their capacities for public health surveillance and response. The regulations were updated in response to the crisis resulting from the Severe Acute Respiratory Syndrome (SARS) epidemic in 2003 in Asia and concerns about circulating Influenza A (H5N1) (sometimes called 'avian flu'). The regulations require countries to strengthen their capacities for public health surveillance and response. The Global Outbreak Alert and Response Network (GOARN) was initiated in 2000 as a technical collaboration to pool human and technical resources for rapid identification, confirmation and response to outbreaks of international importance (World Health Organization 2011a).

The new regulations and network were first tested when an outbreak of Influenza A (H1N1) (sometimes called 'swine flu') was reported to the WHO from Mexico and the USA in April 2009. It was categorized as a 'public health emergency of international concern' and scientific and epidemiological investigations followed, with unprecedented sharing of information between collaborating institutions (Schuchat et al. 2011), member states and the WHO. The WHO coordinated surveillance of cases and eventually classified it as a **pandemic** on the basis of outbreaks in countries from different WHO regions. While the extent of the 2009 pandemic was not as great as originally feared, it is difficult to evaluate to what extent this was the result of the early detection, response and control efforts undertaken in several countries and the efforts coordinated by the WHO. This highlights the important role of surveillance both at the national and international level.

Activity 12.1

Acute lower respiratory infections (ALRI – pneumonia and bronchitis) are a leading cause of illness and mortality in children under 5 years of age in low-income countries. Country X set up a hospital-based surveillance of clinically diagnosed ALRIs in 2004, using five sentinel hospitals. Figure 12.5 shows data from the first five years of surveillance.

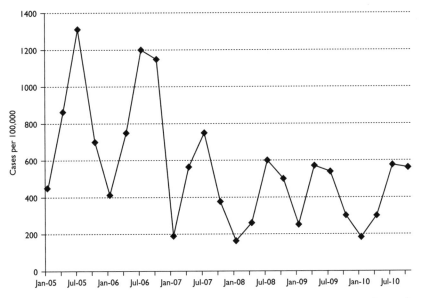

Figure 12.5 Incidence of acute lower respiratory tract infections per 100,000 cases by 3-month reporting period

Source: Ilona Carneiro.

1 Describe the data shown in Figure 12.5.
2 What are the potential biases of these data for:
(a) planning hospital-based ALRI healthcare for Country X?
(b) estimating the true burden of ALRI disease in Country X?

Activity 12.2

1 Nosocomial (i.e. hospital-acquired) infections are an increasing problem in high-income countries. Hospitals with low rates of nosocomial infection tend to have strong infection-control programmes. Two methods of hospital surveillance of post-surgery nosocomial infections were compared in several hospitals in a high-income country. Passive surveillance (clinically diagnosed infections by the surgeon) was

found to have 65% sensitivity and 98% specificity when compared with active surveillance (retrospective review of hospital records and discharge notes by trained medical personnel). What are the benefits and disadvantages of setting up an active surveillance system for nosocomial infections in this setting?

2 Rift Valley Fever (RVF) is a mosquito-borne viral zoonosis (i.e. it can be transmitted from animals to humans). RVF outbreaks have been reported regularly in Sub-Saharan and North Africa since 2006, and are usually preceded by high rates of abortion among sheep and goats. Most human infections have mild influenza-like symptoms, but RVF can cause more severe symptoms including haemorrhagic fever and death. In 2011, after several cases were confirmed by laboratory testing, an epidemiological surveillance network for RVF was set up in a low-income African country. What are the benefits and limitations of using a passive surveillance system that provides reporting forms to village health workers with monthly collection of data?

Monitoring and evaluation

Epidemiology has an important role in health programme monitoring and evaluation. Monitoring is the term applied to the systematic routine collection of evidence about the effectiveness of a specific health programme over a period of time. It involves the collection of descriptive data to ensure that programmes will meet their goals. Epidemiological data used for monitoring include measures of outcome frequency (i.e. prevalence, risk, incidence rate), indicators related to the outcome of interest (e.g. anaemia prevalence as an indicator of impact on malaria), and data on adverse events.

Data on adverse events are a type of outcome measure that must be collected when a clinical intervention (e.g. medication, vaccine, X-ray) is being applied to a population. While an intervention must have been demonstrated as safe before it can be implemented, few intervention studies would have sufficient statistical power to detect rare events. Adverse events that may not have been detected during a Phase 3 trial may become apparent once an intervention is applied to larger populations, under routine conditions (i.e. poorer compliance or clinical follow-up), and over longer periods of time. These are sometimes referred to as Phase 4 studies.

Monitoring often involves measuring process indicators in relation to pre-specified targets. This may be numbers of cases detected by a screening programme, numbers of hospital admissions or waiting times for surgical interventions. Coverage is a measure of what proportion of the eligible population is reached by the intervention (e.g. proportion of children under 12 months old receiving three doses of diphtheria-tetanus-pertussis vaccine, proportion of births attended by a skilled-birth attendant).

For a complex intervention, each step necessary for effective delivery should be monitored. For example, the success of a vaccination programme will depend on: (a) the acquisition of a quality-controlled vaccine; (b) delivery of viable vaccine to health centres; (c) sufficient training of health workers on vaccination; (d) availability of viable vaccine, disposable needles and syringes at the time of attendance; (e) attendance of infants for vaccination; and finally (f) the protection of the infant by the vaccine. Monitoring may therefore measure several essential and desirable indicators along a programme's *process pathway*.

Monitoring may make use of indicators that are collected routinely as part of a country's health information system or indicators introduced as part of a specific health programme. The equity of a programme can also be measured by comparing process indicators across groups, for example, using household income quintiles (i.e. dividing the population at risk into five equal-sized groups based on their income).

Outcome indicators can be collected using cross-sectional or cohort methods, or more often may be collected routinely through passive surveillance or health-facility data. Process indicators can be collected routinely, through the development or adaptation of existing data collection tools. For example, a child health card may be revised to include an additional space for a new vaccination that has been introduced, and the vaccination clinic records will be similarly adapted.

To measure coverage or differential access to a health programme, surveys of a representative sample of those at risk can be conducted. For example, routine data from a mother and child clinic may indicate that all infants attending received their measles vaccinations. If we have a good estimate of the number of infants in the community, we can calculate coverage. Otherwise a household survey may provide more accurate data on *which* households are not sending their children for vaccination, and *why*. This information can be used to improve coverage or equity.

Evaluation is taken here to mean the measurement of a programme's effects and effectiveness after a specified time-period. Note that healthcare evaluation is a broad field, and evaluation can involve needs assessment and cost-effectiveness, for example, which will not be covered here. The *effect* of a programme refers to whether it has achieved delivery of the public health intervention or service and is usually measured by coverage e.g. proportion of women over 50 attending for a regular mammogram.

The *effectiveness* of a programme refers to whether it has had a measurable public health impact in terms of improving health outcomes (e.g. decline in chicken pox (*Varicella zoster*) incidence after the introduction of the varicella vaccine). Process and outcome data can be compared to assess whether the health programme has had any result. A vaccination programme could not claim responsibility for substantial declines in disease-specific child mortality if insufficient stocks of vaccine had been delivered to vaccination clinics, and the number of children receiving the vaccine had been very low. If there are sufficient data points (e.g. from several time-points or sub-populations), a simple analysis might compare process indicators with outcome measures, using a scatter plot (Chapter 5).

Plausibility studies (see Chapter 10) may be used to estimate effectiveness by comparing outcome frequency in the population before and after introduction of the programme; comparing a population covered by the programme with a population without access to the programme; or comparing individuals who did and did not receive a particular type of public health intervention or healthcare. For example, this could include mortality rates among those with short versus long diagnosis-to-treatment intervals, using a pre-defined cut-off. Case-control studies may provide a more rapid means of assessing effectiveness, although they will be subject to different biases (see Chapter 8). For example, cases of *Haemophilous influenzae* type b (Hib) identified from notifiable disease surveillance systems could be compared with community age-matched controls to compare the odds of having received routine infant Hib vaccination (from health records).

The documentation of time-trends following introduction of a health programme may provide supportive evidence of its effectiveness. However, for these 'adequacy evaluations' to be convincing, the programme's process pathway needs be relatively short and simple, the impact should be large, and confounding must be unlikely (Victora et al. 2004).

Activity 12.3

This activity is based on the monitoring and evaluation of a malaria intervention programme by Hanson et al. (2008). Pregnant women and children under 5 years of age
are a high-risk group for severe malaria outcomes. Insecticide-treated nets (ITNs)
provide protection from night-biting mosquitoes to those sleeping under them, and
have been proven safe and effective in reducing maternal anaemia and child mortality,
particularly in Africa. A programme was established in Tanzania to increase ITN coverage of pregnant women and young children through the delivery of vouchers during
the first antenatal care (ANC) visit. Vouchers provided a subsidy (i.e. price reduction)
for purchasing an ITN in local shops.

Suppose you are part of a team involved in designing a monitoring and evaluation
strategy for this complex intervention.

1 Identify the intermediary processes involved in achieving the programme's aims.
2 Which process indicators and methods would you use to monitor how well the
  programme was functioning and whether it was on track to deliver its outputs?
3 Describe how you would evaluate the effectiveness of the programme after a
  five-year period. Identify the primary outcome measure and methods for collecting
  relevant data.

Informing policy and practice

While epidemiology aims to influence public health policy and practice, decision-
makers often need to act rapidly and, if evidence is incomplete or contradictory, may
do so in the absence of good evidence. The results of epidemiological studies, and
routine data on the burden of an outcome or risk of an exposure, need to be
communicated appropriately and rapidly to policy-makers.

An example of poor medical research data having a detrimental impact on public
health is the controversy over claims that measles–mumps–rubella (MMR) vaccine
caused autism. In 1998, a study of 12 children with developmental disorders reported
that parents of eight of these children linked the start of behavioural symptoms to recent
MMR vaccination (Wakefield et al. 1998). No further epidemiological evidence was presented, but high profile media coverage led to a significant decline in MMR coverage in
the UK. Concerned parents refused to vaccinate their children, and increases in the
numbers of confirmed measles cases followed. Subsequent epidemiological research,
including a large case-control study using routine data from general practitioners (Smeeth
et al. 2004), found no association between MMR vaccination and autism. However, these
took time to conduct, analyse and disseminate. MMR coverage in the UK started to
increase after 2003, but by 2011 had still not regained its pre-vaccination-scare level.

Routine monitoring data can inform public health practice through the detection of
and rapid response to outbreaks, and through the detection of more gradual changes
in population health over time. Routine data can also be used to identify risk factors
for subsequent epidemiological investigation. An example of this is the initiation of a
surveillance system for AIDS soon after it was first described, which subsequently
provided data that helped to identify high-risk groups and risk factors for the disease,
long before its cause was discovered.

Epidemiological research data have often been used successfully to inform public
health policy and practice. Examples include national policies on routine childhood

vaccination to prevent specific childhood infectious diseases, and public policies and legislation to reduce exposure to tobacco smoke. Epidemiological evidence that obesity is caused by complex interactions between diet and physical activity is currently informing the development of policies to slow the obesity epidemic in high-income countries. In the UK, for example, the government is attempting a controversial health promotion approach to encourage individual behaviour change.

The importance of collecting high quality data increases as data access and usage grow. As more agencies and individuals, including policy-makers and the media, have access to descriptive information on the health of populations its use (and misuse) will increase. We hope that reading this book has given you the incentive and basic tools to collect, analyse, or interpret public health data using effective epidemiological tools.

Conclusion

In this chapter you have learned about surveillance, monitoring and evaluation for public health. Epidemiological methods, rigour and analysis can be applied to routinely collected data to continually inform public health policy and practice. Surveillance systems allow us to identify disease outbreaks and epidemics, monitor time trends and identify population-level risk factors for an outcome. Demographic systems (i.e. vital registration, population census) provide contextual baseline and denominator data within which monitoring can be interpreted. Routine monitoring of process and outcome indicators can be used to evaluate the impact of public health programmes. Epidemiological data from research and routine monitoring can be used to provide an evidence-base for making informed public health decisions.

References

Centers for Disease Control and Prevention (2004) Summary of notifiable diseases—United States, 2002. *Morbidity Mortality Weekly Report* 51: 1–84.

Centers for Disease Control and Prevention (2009) Estimated county-level prevalence of diabetes and obesity—United States, 2007. *Morbidity Mortality Weekly Report* 58: 1259–63.

Centers for Disease Control and Prevention (2010) Summary of Notifiable Diseases—United States, 2008. *Morbidity Mortality Weekly Report* 57: 1–94.

Hanson K, Nathan R, Marchant T, et al. (2008) Vouchers for scaling up insecticide-treated nets in Tanzania: methods for monitoring and evaluation of a national health system intervention. *BMC Public Health* 8: 205.

Jones C, Abeku TA, Rapuoda B, Okia M and Cox J (2008) District-based malaria epidemic early warning systems in East Africa: perceptions of acceptability and usefulness among key staff at health facility, district and central levels. *Social Science and Medicine* 67(2): 292–300.

Schuchat A, Bell BP and Redd SC (2011) The science behind preparing and responding to pandemic influenza: the lessons and limits of science. *Clinical Infectious Diseases* 52 Suppl. 1: S8–12.

Smeeth L, Cook C, Fombonne E, et al. (2004) MMR vaccination and pervasive developmental disorders: a case-control study. *Lancet* 364: 963–9.

Victora CG, Habicht JP and Bryce J (2004) Evidence-based public health: moving beyond randomized trials. *American Journal of Public Health* 94: 400–5.

Wakefield AJ, Murch SH, Anthony A, et al. (1998) Ileal-lymphoid-nodular hyperplasia, non-specific colitis, and pervasive developmental disorder in children. *Lancet* 351: 637–41.

World Health Organization (2011a) *Global Outbreak Alert and Response* [Online]. Available: http://www.who.int/csr/en/ (accessed 02/05/2011).

World Health Organization (2011b) *International Health Regulations (IHR)* [Online]. Available: http://www. who.int/ihr/global_alert/en/ (accessed 02/05/2011).

Feedback on activities

Activity 12.1

Your answers should be similar to the following.

1 The data show an annual seasonal variation in the incidence of ALRI, with peaks in July–September, and lows in January–March. There appears to be a halving of the incidence between 2006 and 2007, which is then sustained for the subsequent three years. The peak incidence declines from approximately 1,200 cases per 10,000 (2005 and 2006) to approximately 600 cases per 100,000 (2007–2010), while the low incidence declines from approximately 400 per 100,000 (2005 and 2006) to 200 per 100,000 (2007–2010).

Without more historical data, we cannot tell whether the 2005–2006 data represent unusual or epidemic incidence, or whether these data represent a stable incidence with a subsequent decline, for example, after the introduction of a public health intervention.

2 These data present biases at two levels:

(a) The data may not be representative of other hospitals in country X because they come from five sentinel hospitals. This can result in selection bias if the geographical location of the sentinel hospitals is not nationally representative. For example, they may be more likely to be in urban rather than rural settings, in additional to potential regional and ethnic differences. Sentinel hospitals also tend to be chosen because they have sufficient capacity for diagnosis and reporting, which is likely to vary from the infrastructure in most other hospitals.

(b) In addition to the reasons given above relating to geographical and social representativeness of the sentinel hospitals, hospital or health-facility-based data generally underestimate the community burden of most diseases. Many people may not access government healthcare services because of distance, poor quality of care (perceived or real), economics (e.g. in settings with cost-sharing, travel costs), or social exclusion. There are also likely to be several alternative sources of healthcare (e.g. mission hospitals, private and traditional practitioners).

As these are designated sentinel hospitals, the quality of data are likely to be monitored and of a reasonable standard. However, a large number of staff will be involved, and there may be differences in diagnosis and reporting within and between sites, and over time.

Activity 12.2

1 Active surveillance is very costly, taking time and requiring additional staff.

However, a sensitivity of 65% means that 100 − 65 = 35% of patients with nosocomial infections were not being identified by the surgeon, i.e. the rate of nosocomial infections was being underestimated. If the surgeons and the hospital are unaware of the magnitude of the problem, it is unlikely to be resolved.

An active surveillance system would therefore most probably result in better recognition of the burden of nosocomial infections, and subsequent improvements in infection control. As retrospective review does not impact patient care it may be preferable to set up a sample active surveillance, with retrospective review of a randomly selected proportion of patients as an indicator of the problem.

2 Routine monitoring by personnel with limited training is unlikely to provide accurate or comparable data. However, this surveillance aims to detect outbreaks, rather than routinely 'monitor' for secular trends or to compare populations, therefore data consistency is not the top priority. The most important issue here will be high coverage, which would not be possible with an active surveillance system.

As RVF outbreaks are generally preceded by high rates of abortion among livestock, resident village health workers will be best placed to detect these warning signs. Since the majority of cases have non-specific symptoms, active surveillance would be unable to rely on clinical diagnosis anyway, and laboratory facilities are unlikely to be routinely available.

Collation of monthly reports can be used to 'screen' for areas with increasing numbers of reported influenza-like cases for further investigation. Any reports of cases with more severe symptoms that had not already been notified through the formal healthcare system, would identify the local population as high-risk. (A cross-sectional serological survey (i.e. testing antibody levels) could then be conducted.)

Activity 12.3

1 The intermediary processes can be identified as:
- Vouchers available in health facilities.
- Pregnant women attending for routine antenatal care (ANC) visits.
- Pregnant women receiving a subsidy voucher.
- Pregnant women seeking to purchase an ITN.
- ITNs available for purchase with the voucher in the local shops.
- Pregnant women sleeping under an ITN.
- Babies or young children co-sleeping under an ITN.

2 Appropriate process indicators for monitoring should correspond to each of the intermediary processes. You may have identified some or all of the following.
- Health facility stock records could be used to document receipt and availability of subsidy vouchers.
- Health facility records could provide information on the number of women attending for ANC, and demographic data can be used to estimate the number of pregnant women in the population.
- Pregnant women could be interviewed as they leave the health facility ANC clinic to evaluate what proportion were given a voucher by the health facility staff. This is known as an 'exit interview'. These data could also be obtained from a cross-sectional household survey.
- A household survey might ask about the willingness to purchase a net given that there is some cost to the household. This is a complex issue involving household economics and decision-making powers, and would probably require additional qualitative methods.
- A structured interview administered to a random sample of shopkeepers could collect data on ITN availability in the local shops, and participation of shops in the voucher programme. This is known as a 'retail audit' and could be undertaken at regular intervals. Additional qualitative data on shopkeeper perceptions of the voucher scheme, collected through in-depth interviews, could identify potential difficulties.

- Routine programme records on the exchange of vouchers for financial subsidy by shopkeepers could be used to monitor how the process was functioning.
- A cross-sectional household survey could be used to measure the effects of the programme. The main effects of interest would be the proportion of households with a pregnant woman that own an ITN, the proportion of pregnant women reporting that they regularly sleep under an ITN, and the proportion of infants or young children reported to regularly sleep under an ITN.

3 While the aim of the programme is 'to increase ITN coverage of pregnant women and young children', its ultimate goal is to reduce adverse malaria outcomes in this high-risk target group:

- Child mortality would be hard to measure, and would have to rely on demographic data such as population censuses or representative population surveys, which may not take place within the five-year time-period.
- Maternal anaemia would be the preferred outcome measure as it could be measured at routine ANC visits. This would not require many additional resources, as training and strengthening of data recording systems would already be implemented in the health facilities and ANC clinics as part of the programme.
- Maternal anaemia is related to low birthweight, but this is harder to measure in a developing country setting as a low proportion of births are attended by skilled birth attendants.
- More direct measures of malaria outcome include outpatient attendance for clinical malaria, or hospital admissions for severe malaria. However, these data would be dependent on the quality of data collection at the hospitals or health facilities.

Glossary

This is a reference guide to the epidemiological terms used in this book. For further explanation of these terms, use the index to refer to them in the main text. Cross-references to other glossary terms are shown in italics.

Absolute risk See *attributable risk*.

Active surveillance The *surveillance* of an *outcome* by searching for *cases* in the community.

Allocation The distribution of study subjects to *intervention* and *control* arms in an *intervention study*.

Allocation concealment In a *randomized-controlled trial*: when the *randomization* schedule for *intervention* allocation is not revealed to the person enrolling subjects, to reduce *selection bias*.

Alternative hypothesis Usually the opposite of the *null hypothesis*, but may indicate the direction of an association.

Analytical study Designed to test a *hypothesis*. Generally, to examine whether a certain *exposure* is a *risk factor* for a particular *outcome*. (Contrast: *descriptive*.)

Ascertainment bias A type of *information bias*, where detection of *outcome* may vary between *exposure* groups. May be especially a problem for *intervention studies* without *blinding*.

Assessment bias See *information bias*.

Asymptomatic The state of having an *outcome* with no outward *symptoms*.

Attributable fraction (Synonym: Attributable risk percentage.) A measure that calculates the *attributable risk* as a *proportion* of the incidence of *outcome* in those *exposed*, i.e. the proportion of *cases* among those exposed that may be due to the *exposure*, and that could be prevented if the exposure were eliminated completely.

Attributable risk (Synonym: *absolute risk, excess risk*.) A measure that calculates the additional incidence of *outcome* in those *exposed* after subtracting the incidence that would have occurred in the absence of *exposure* (i.e. in those *unexposed*). It assumes that the relationship between exposure and outcome is causal, and can be calculated using either *risks* or *incidence rates*. It is used to indicate the number of *cases* that could be prevented if the exposure were eliminated completely, i.e. the public health impact.

Attributable risk percentage See *attributable fraction*.

Bias A *systematic* difference from the truth. In epidemiology, this represents a source of error in estimating the association between *exposure* and *outcome*. (See *selection bias, information bias*.)

Blinding (Synonym: masking.) Where information about *exposure* or *outcome* is concealed from the participants and/or observers to reduce *information bias*.

Case An individual that meets the *case definition* for having the *outcome* of interest.

Case-control study An *observational study* in which two groups are defined on the basis of their *outcome* status. Those with the outcome are called *cases* and those without the outcome are called *controls*. The level of *exposure* to a *risk factor* is then measured in the two groups and compared. The *odds ratio of exposure* is the only measure of *relative risk* that can be obtained from case-control studies, as there is no measure of the *frequency* of the outcome.

Case definition Criteria for identifying an individual as having the health outcome of interest, which may specify clinical signs and symptoms, diagnostic test results and time-period (e.g. a malaria case as malaria bloodslide positive with reported fever within 48 hours).

Case-fatality rate The *proportion* of cases with an *outcome*, which are fatal within a specified period of time. (Note, this is a *proportion* not a *rate*.)

Causal pathway The sequence of events leading from an *exposure* to an *outcome*.

Causality The relationship between an *exposure* and a health *outcome*, where the outcome is considered to be a consequence of the exposure.

Chance The possibility of observing a value or event without reason or predictability. In epidemiology this is often taken to mean that something is not representative of the reality.

Cluster-randomized trial A *randomized-controlled trial* in which groups of individuals (clusters) rather than single individuals are *randomized*, and all individuals within a cluster receive the same *intervention*.

Cohort study (Synonym: follow-up study.) An *observational study* in which two groups are defined on the basis of their *exposure* to a potential *risk factor*, and are followed up over time to measure the *incidence* of the *outcome*, which is then compared between the groups to give an estimate of *relative risk*.

Compliance rate In an *intervention study*: the *proportion* of individuals who cooperate fully with all the study procedures. (Note, this is a *proportion* not a *rate*.)

Component cause A factor that contributes to producing an outcome.

Confidence interval The range of values, estimated from a *sample*, within which the 'true' *population* value is likely to be found. A 95 per cent confidence interval is usually presented, meaning that there is a 5 per cent probability that the 'true' *population* value lies outside of this range. It is used to indicate the reliability of the estimated result.

Confounder (Synonym: *confounding* variable.) A variable that is associated with both the *exposure* and the *outcome* under study, but is not on the causal pathway between the two. It may provide an alternative explanation for any association observed.

Confounding A situation in which the estimate of association between an *exposure* and an *outcome* is distorted because of the association of the exposure with another factor (see *confounder*) that is also associated with the *outcome*.

Consent See *informed consent*.

Contamination In an *intervention study*: exposure of the *control* group to the *intervention*, or vice versa.

Control (Case-control) An individual that does not fulfil the *case definition* for the outcome of interest. (Contrast: *case*.) Note, this is different to the meaning of *control* in an *intervention* study.

Control (Intervention) A study subject (individual, household, village, etc.) in an *intervention study* who does not receive, and is therefore *unexposed* to, the *intervention* of interest. Note, this is different to the meaning in a *case-control* study.

Cross-sectional study An *observational study* in which information on the *outcome* and *exposure* is measured simultaneously (at one point in time).

Crossover trial A *randomized-controlled trial* in which each subject acts as its own control by receiving both the *intervention* and *control* at different time-points, with a *washout period* in-between.

Crude rate The *incidence rate* in the total *population*, without any adjustment for potential confounders. (Contrast: *standardized rate*.)

Cumulative incidence See *risk*.

Descriptive Designed to describe the existing distribution of variables in a *population* without regard to *causal* or other associations. An example would be a *cross-sectional study* to assess the *prevalence* of anaemia in a population. (Contrast: *analytical study*.)

Diagnosis Identification of an *outcome* using rigorous tests or methods.

Differential misclassification Incorrect classification of *exposure* or *outcome* of study subjects as a result of *information bias*, where this differs between comparison groups. This can lead to over- or under-estimation of a measure of association and may lead to false associations.

Direct standardization See *standardization*.

Ecological bias (Synonym: *ecological fallacy*.)

Ecological fallacy (Synonym: *ecological bias*.) The misleading idea that a group-level association from an *ecological study* can be applied at the individual level. For example, a positive correlation between national average dietary fat intake and national mortality rates from female breast cancer does not necessarily mean that the women who died of breast cancer were the ones who had a diet rich in fat.

Ecological study An *observational study* in which the units of analysis are populations or groups of people rather than individuals. (See *ecological fallacy*.)

Effect modification (Synonym: *interaction*.) Variation in effect of the *exposure* on an *outcome* across values of another factor (*effect modifier*). It can be detected by *stratification* during analysis and may be adjusted for with *statistical modelling*.

Effect modifier Factor across whose categories the effect of an *exposure* on particular *outcome* may vary. See *effect modification*.

Effectiveness The extent to which an *intervention* produces an improvement in a health *outcome* when it is applied through a routine delivery system. (Contrast: *efficacy*.)

Efficacy The extent to which an *intervention* produces an improvement in a health *outcome* under ideal trial conditions. (Contrast: *effectiveness*.)

Elimination The total removal of an *outcome* (usually by removal of the *exposure*) from a country or region. (Contrast: *eradication*.)

Endemic The maintenance of an infection in a defined *population* without external introduction.

Epidemic The increase in the *frequency* of an *outcome* that is significantly in excess of what would normally be expected.

Eradication The total removal of an *outcome* (usually by removal of the *exposure*) from the entire world. (Contrast: *elimination*.)

Excess risk See *attributable risk*.

Exclusion criteria Characteristics defining which individuals may not be included in a study. (Contrast: *inclusion criteria*.)

Exposed Those subjects who have experienced or possess (e.g. genetic or physical characteristics) the *risk factor* of interest.

Exposure Synonymous with *risk factor*, or the act of being exposed to a potential risk or *protective factor*.

Factorial trial A *randomized-controlled trial* in which two or more *interventions* are compared individually and in combination against a *control* comparison group.

Follow-up Observation over a period of time of an individual, group, or initially defined population whose relevant characteristics have been assessed, in order to observe changes in *exposures* or *outcomes*.

Frequency A measure of the number of occurrences of an outcome per *population* (see *prevalence*) or per unit time (see *incidence*).

General population The wider population to whom the results of analytical epidemiological studies are to be applied. For example, the 'general population of India' refers to all individuals living in India. (Contrast: *sample population, target population*.)

Hypothesis A supposition phrased in such a way as to allow it to be tested and confirmed or refuted.

Incidence The number of new *cases* of an *outcome* that develop in a defined *population* of individuals at risk during a specified period of time. It can be measured as *risk, odds* or *incidence rate*. See *null hypothesis*.

Incidence rate The number of new *cases* of an *outcome* that develop in a defined *population* of individuals at risk during a specified period of time, divided by the total *person-time at risk*.

Incidence rate ratio (Synonym: *rate ratio*.) A measure of *relative risk*. Calculated as the *incidence rate* of outcome in those exposed, divided by the incidence rate of outcome in those unexposed.

Inclusion criteria Characteristics defining which individuals may be included in a study. (Contrast: *exclusion criteria*.)

Indirect standardization See *standardization*.

Information bias (Synonym: *measurement bias, assessment bias*.) Error due to *systematic* differences in the measurement or classification of study participants. See *observer bias, responder bias, misclassification*.

Informed consent Voluntary agreement to participate in an epidemiological study after receiving sufficient details of the aims, methods, and potential risks and benefits of the study.

Intention-to-treat analysis In *intervention studies*: subjects are analysed on the basis of initial *intervention allocation* irrespective of whether they complied with this allocation.

Interaction See *effect modification*.

Interim analysis Independent analysis of a *randomized-controlled trial* before the planned finish in the case of safety concerns or lack of study *power* to detect an effect.

Intervention The preventive or therapeutic measure under study in an *intervention study*. Also refers to medical or public health involvement to change the developmental process of an *outcome*.

Intervention efficacy A measure of the proportion of incidence of an *outcome* that can be prevented by an *intervention*. See also *protective efficacy*.

Intervention study *Analytical* study designed to test whether there is a causal relationship by reducing/removing exposure to a *risk factor*, or increasing/introducing exposure to a *protective factor*, and observing the effect on the *outcome*. *Randomized-controlled trial* is an example of an intervention study design. (Contrast: *observational study*.)

Latent Time between acquiring an *outcome* and appearance of *symptoms*.

Lead-time bias A type of *bias* resulting from the time difference between detection of an *outcome* or *risk factor*, and the appearance of symptoms, that may lead to an apparent increase in survival time even if there is no effect on the outcome.

Length-time bias A type of *bias* resulting from differences in the length of time taken for an *outcome* to progress to severe effects, that may affect the apparent *efficacy* of a *screening* method.

Masking See *blinding.*

Matching A technique used to control for *confounding* during study design. The comparison groups are selected to have the same distribution of potential confounders by matching individually (pair matching) or at a group-level (frequency matching).

Measurement bias See *information bias.*

Minimization Method of *allocation* that aims to minimize differences between the *intervention* and *control* arms in a small *randomized-controlled trial* where there may be several *confounders* or *effect modifiers.*

Necessary cause A *component cause* that is essential for an outcome to occur.

Negative predictive value The proportion of individuals identified as not having an *outcome* by a *screening* or diagnostic method that truly do not have the outcome. See *positive predictive value, screening, sensitivity, specificity.*

Nested case-control study *Case-control study* where *cases* and *controls* are identified from a *prospective cohort* study, reducing problems of *information bias.*

Non-differential misclassification Incorrect classification of *exposure* or *outcome* of study subjects as a result of *information bias,* where this does not vary between comparison groups. This can lead to an underestimation of the strength (statistical significance) of an association.

Notifiable disease A disease that is required by law to be reported to government authorities to enable national *surveillance.*

Null hypothesis A falsifiable *hypothesis* against which to statistically test data. Usually, that there is no association between an exposure and outcome. (Contrast: *alternative hypothesis.*)

Observational study *Analytical* study in which the role of the investigator is to observe the relationship between an *exposure* and *outcome. Ecological, cross-sectional, cohort* and *case-control* are examples of observational study designs. (Contrast: *intervention study.*)

Observer bias *Information bias* introduced by those measuring or assessing the *outcome.*

Occupational cohort A group of individuals selected for *prospective* study on the basis of a shared occupation.

Odds (of exposure) The number of individuals in a defined *population* exposed to a particular *risk factor,* divided by the number of individuals not exposed to that risk factor in the same *population.*

Odds (of outcome) The number of new *cases* of an *outcome* that develop in a defined *population* of individuals at risk during a specified period of time, divided by the number of individuals who do not develop the outcome during the same time-period. It can be interpreted as the ratio of the *risk* that the outcome will occur to the risk that it will not occur during a specified period of time.

Odds ratio (of exposure) Calculated as the *odds* of *exposure* in those with the outcome, divided by the odds of exposure in those without the outcome. Used in *case-control studies* as an estimate of the *relative risk,* because incidence cannot be measured.

Odds ratio (of outcome) A measure of *relative risk.* Calculated as the *odds* of *outcome* in those exposed, divided by the odds of outcome in those unexposed.

Outbreak A sudden *epidemic,* usually of short duration. See *epidemic.*

Outcome A health state or event of interest such as infection, illness, disability, or death, or a health indicator such as high blood pressure or presence of antibodies. Can also be specified as the opposite of any of these.

Overmatching In a *case-control study*: where *matching* results in *cases* and *controls* that are too similar with respect to the *exposure* of interest to enable detection of an association with *outcome*.

P-value The numerical probability that an observed value or estimated association from a *sample* occurred by chance alone, and that it does not exist in the *population* from which the sample was selected.

Pandemic An *epidemic* that is occurring in populations over a large number of countries or worldwide.

Passive surveillance The *surveillance* of an *outcome* by detection of *cases* when they seek healthcare.

Per-protocol analysis In *intervention studies*: subjects are analysed on the basis of actual compliance with initial *intervention allocation*.

Period prevalence The number of existing *cases* of an *outcome* in a defined *population* during a specified (short) period of time divided by the total number of people in that *population* during the same time-period. It is a *proportion*.

Person-time at risk The sum of the time each individual in a defined population is at risk of an *outcome*. It is used as a denominator in the calculation of *incidence rates*.

Pilot study A small-scale study conducted prior to the main study to test methods, data collection, data entry, etc.

Placebo An inert medication or procedure that may be given to the *control* group in an *intervention trial*, specified as a placebo-controlled trial.

Plausibility studies A type of *intervention study* designed to examine whether an *intervention might reasonably be considered* to reduce a particular *outcome*. Due to practical or ethical limitations, the methods for reducing the effects of *chance*, *bias* and *confounding* are not as rigorous as with a *randomized-controlled trial*. Mostly used to evaluate the *effectiveness* of an intervention or healthcare programme.

Point prevalence (Synonym: *prevalence*.) The number of existing *cases* of an *outcome* in a defined *population* at a particular point in time divided by the total number of people in that *population* at the same time. It is a *proportion*.

Population Individuals with a shared characteristic (usually geographic area). See *general population, sample population, target population*.

Population attributable fraction (Synonym: *population attributable risk percentage*.) A measure that calculates the *population attributable risk* as a proportion of the incidence of *outcome* in the population, i.e. the proportion of *cases* in the population that may be due to the *exposure*, and that could be prevented if the exposure were eliminated completely.

Population attributable risk A measure that calculates the additional incidence of *outcome* in the population after subtracting the incidence that would have occurred in the absence of *exposure* (i.e. in those *unexposed*). (See also *attributable risk*.)

Population attributable risk percentage See *population attributable fraction*.

Positive predictive value The proportion of individuals identified as having an *outcome* by a *screening* or diagnostic method that truly have the outcome. See *negative predictive value, screening, sensitivity, specificity*.

Power The statistical probability of detecting an association if it is real.

Precision The statistical probability of detecting an association by chance (i.e. if it is not real).

Prevalence See *point prevalence* and *period prevalence*.

Prevalence ratio An estimate of the magnitude of association between *exposure* and *prevalence* of an *outcome*. Calculated as the prevalence of outcome in those exposed to a particular *risk factor*, divided by the prevalence of outcome in those unexposed.

Preventable fraction A measure that calculates the additional incidence of *outcome* in those *unexposed* to a *protective factor* after subtracting the incidence that would have occurred in the presence of *exposure* (i.e. in those *exposed*). It is calculated by subtracting the relative risk from 1. (Contrast: *attributable fraction*.) See also *protective efficacy*.

Prevention paradox The concept that a large reduction in *exposure* among a few individuals at high risk of an *outcome* may not have as great an impact at the population-level as a slight reduction in exposure by many individuals.

Primary prevention *Intervention* to prevent the onset of an *outcome* by removing or reducing *exposure*. (Contrast: *secondary prevention, tertiary prevention*.)

Prognosis A medical term used to describe the likely end result (e.g. survival, recovery) of an *outcome*.

Proportion The relationship between two numbers of the same type where one is a part and the other the whole. By definition, it can only take values between 0 and 1 (or between 0 per cent and 100 per cent if expressed as a percentage). See *prevalence, risk*.

Prospective cohort *Cohort study* in which on-going data collection enables measurement of *incidence* after exposure has been recorded. (Contrast: *retrospective cohort*.)

Protective efficacy A measure of the proportion of incidence of an *outcome* that can be prevented by a *protective factor*. See also *preventable fraction*.

Protective factor (Synonym: protective *risk factor*.) A *risk factor* that is associated with a decreased probability of a negative health *outcome*. (Contrast: *risk factor*.)

Random allocation See *randomization*.

Random error The variation of an observed *sample* value from the true *population* value due to *chance* alone.

Random selection Selection in a random (unpredictable) manner where each study unit (person, village, school) has an equal (or known) probability of being selected.

Randomization Where allocation to *intervention* groups is determined by chance, i.e. each study unit has the same probability of being allocated to each of the intervention groups, and the probability that a given unit will receive a particular intervention is independent of the probability that any other unit will receive the same intervention. (See *randomized controlled trial*.)

Randomized-controlled trial An *intervention study* in which the *intervention* is compared to a *control*, and allocation of intervention is by *randomization*.

Rate The relationship between two numbers of different types. In epidemiology it refers to the occurrence of events per unit time. See *incidence rate*.

Rate difference See *attributable risk*.

Rate ratio See *incidence rate ratio*.

Ratio The relationship between two numbers of the same type, either expressed as a:b or a/b. See *prevalence ratio, risk ratio, odds ratio, incidence rate ratio, standardized mortality ratio*.

Reference category The group against which all others are compared. This is usually the *unexposed* group.

Regression *Statistical modelling* to explain how much variation in one variable may be the result of other variables. It enables us to estimate the association between *exposure* and *outcome*, adjusting for the effects of *confounding* and *effect modification*.

Relative risk An estimate of the magnitude of association between *exposure* and incidence of an *outcome*. It can be interpreted as the likelihood of developing an *outcome* in those exposed compared to those unexposed. It can be calculated as *risk ratio, odds ratio* and *incidence rate ratio*.

Representative sample A *sample* that has the same characteristics as the *population* from which it was selected.

Residual confounding The effects of *confounding* that remain even after adjustment because data on the *confounder* are not sufficiently accurate.

Responder bias *Information bias* introduced by study participants, or those providing relevant information on study participants.

Restriction A technique used to control for *confounding* during study design. It limits the study to people who are similar in relation to the confounder.

Retrospective cohort *Cohort study* in which historical data are collected and there is no follow-up of study participants. (Contrast: *prospective cohort.*)

Reverse causality A situation in which an apparent *risk factor* may be a consequence of the *outcome*.

Risk (Synonym: *cumulative incidence.*) The number of new *cases* of an *outcome* that develop in a defined *population* of individuals at risk during a specified period of time, divided by the total number of individuals at risk during the same period of time. It is a *proportion* and can be interpreted as the probability that the *outcome* will occur within a specified time.

Risk factor (Synonym: *exposure.*) An environmental (e.g. radiation), socio-economic (e.g. occupation), behavioural (e.g. alcohol consumption), physical (e.g. height) or inherited (e.g. blood group) factor that is associated with an increased probability of a negative health *outcome*. (Contrast: *protective risk factor.*)

Risk ratio A measure of *relative risk*. Calculated as the *risk* of *outcome* in those exposed, divided by the risk of outcome in those unexposed.

Sample A subset of a *population* selected for study.

Sample population *Subjects* selected for epidemiological study from a wider *population*. See *general population*.

Sample size The number of study units (individuals, groups) under study.

Screening The *systematic* detection of an *outcome* or indicators of increased risk for an outcome among apparently healthy people.

Secondary attack rate A specific type of *risk*: the number of new *cases* of an *outcome* that develop among contacts of an initial *case* during a specified period of time, divided by the total number of contacts at risk during the same period of time.

Secondary prevention *Intervention* to prevent the development of adverse health consequences of an established *outcome*. (Contrast: *primary prevention, tertiary prevention.*)

Secular trends Changes in the *frequency* of an *outcome* or *exposure* in a *population* over time that are expected to be long-term.

Selection bias Error due to *systematic* differences in characteristics between the study participants and the *population* from which they are selected, or between the groups being compared within the study.

Sensitivity (Synonym: true positive 'rate'.) The *proportion* of individuals who truly have an *outcome* that are correctly identified by a *screening* or diagnostic method. (Contrast: *specificity*.)

Sentinel surveillance The *surveillance* of an *outcome* by detecting *cases* through designated institutions with quality control of diagnosis and reporting.

Specificity (Synonym: true negative 'rate'.) The *proportion* of individuals who truly do not have an *outcome* that are correctly identified by a *screening* or diagnostic method. (Contrast: *sensitivity*.)

Standard population A *population* with a defined demographic structure.

Standardization (direct) A technique to remove demographic differences between populations so that they may be compared. The direct method applies the category-specific incidence rates of the *study population* to a *standard population* structure.

Standardization (indirect) A technique to remove demographic differences between populations so that they may be compared. The indirect method applies the category-specific incidence rates of a *standard population* to the *study population* structure. This is used to calculate the *standardized mortality* (or *morbidity*) *ratio*.

Standardized mortality/morbidity ratio A comparative measure of the difference in *outcome* incidence between two populations if they had had the same population demographic structure.

Standardized rate The expected incidence rate in a *population* if it had the same demographic structure as another *population* (or standard *population*) enabling comparison of different *populations*. This is obtained by *standardization*. (Contrast: *crude rate*.)

Statistical modelling Definition of the relationship between two variables using mathematical descriptions. See *regression*.

Statistical significance The probability that a result did not occur by chance. See P-*value*.

Stratification The process of separating a *sample* into several sub-samples according to specified criteria. It can be used to control for *confounding* during analysis, or to detect *effect modification*.

Subject An individual or group participating in a study.

Subjects Units of an epidemiological study. These may be, for example, individuals, households, communities, geographical areas, countries.

Sufficient cause A factor or set of factors that inevitably produces the outcome.

Surveillance The monitoring of *outcomes* in a given *population* over time.

Susceptible An individual that is at risk of acquiring the *outcome* of interest. For example, for many infectious diseases to which immunity is acquired, an immune individual is no longer susceptible to infection. This may also apply to individuals with certain genetic characteristics.

Symptoms Changes noticed by a patient that indicate the presence of an adverse health *outcome*.

Systematic Method that is non-random, ordered or organized.

Target population The *population* to which the results of an epidemiological study are to be extrapolated, or to which a public health intervention is to be applied. This may be a subset or the whole of the *general population*.

Tertiary prevention *Intervention* to reduce progression of an established *outcome* and prevent complications or more severe consequences. (Contrast: *primary prevention*, *secondary prevention*.)

True negative rate See *specificity*. Note this is an incorrect usage of the term *rate*.

True positive rate See *sensitivity*. Note this is an incorrect usage of the term *rate*.

Unexposed Those subjects who have not experienced or do not possess (e.g. genetic or physical characteristics) the *risk factor* of interest.

Vaccine efficacy A measure of the proportion of incidence of an *outcome* that can be prevented by administration of a vaccine. See also *protective efficacy*.

Washout period Period after an *intervention* has been removed during which its effect declines.

Index

Page numbers in *italics* refer to figures and tables.

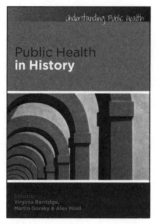

PUBLIC HEALTH IN HISTORY

Virginia Berridge, Martin Gorsky
and Alex Mold

9780335242641 (Paperback)
2011

eBook also available

This fascinating book offers a wide ranging exploration of the history of public health and the development of health services over the past two centuries. The book surveys the rise and redefinition of public health since the sanitary revolution of the mid-nineteenth century, assessing the reforms in the post World War II years and the coming of welfare states.

Written by experts from the London School of Hygiene and Tropical Medicine, this is the definitive history of public health.

Key features:

- Case studies on malaria, sexual health, alcohol and substance abuse
- A comparative examination of why healthcare has taken such different trajectories in different countries
- Exercises enabling readers to easily interact with and critically assess historical source material

www.openup.co.uk

OPEN UNIVERSITY PRESS
McGraw - Hill Education